Diabetes Nursing Care:
Overview and Management

Fourth Edition

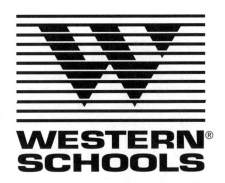

WESTERN® SCHOOLS

By
Sandra Winter, RN, MSN, CDE

WESTERN SCHOOLS

P.O. Box 1930
Brockton, MA 02303
1-800-438-8888

ABOUT THE AUTHOR

Sandra Winter, RN, MSN, CDE, is a diabetes nurse specialist at Scripps Mercy Hospital and Medical Center, San Diego, CA. She has extensive experience in diabetes management, has made many public and professional presentations on diabetes, and has published on the subject of diabetes. She is a member of the American Diabetes Association, Juvenile Diabetes Foundation International, the American Association of Diabetes Educators, and the San Diego Association of Diabetes Educators.

ABOUT THE SUBJECT MATTER EXPERT

Jan L. Lee, RN, PhD, CS, is an Associate Professor and the Director of Undergraduate and Non-Traditional Programs at the University of Michigan School of Nursing, Ann Arbor, MI. Dr. Lee has been funded by the National Institutes of Health to study self-management of diabetes. In addition, she is a consultant to the RAND Corporation, Santa Monica, CA on the quality of nursing care studies. She is a biographee in *Who's Who in Nursing* and *Who's Who in Medicine and Healthcare.*

Subject Matter Expert: Jan L. Lee, RN, PhD, CS

Copy Editor: Diana Melancon, MSN, RN

Indexer: Sylvia Coates

Typesetter: Kathy Johnson

ISBN: 1-57801-033-0

IMPORTANT: Read these instructions *BEFORE* proceeding!

Enclosed with your course book you will find the FasTrax® answer sheet. Use this form to answer all the final exam questions that appear in this course book. If you are completing more than one course, be sure to write your answers on the appropriate answer sheet. Full instructions and complete grading details are printed on the FasTrax instruction sheet, also enclosed with your order. Please review them before starting. *If you are mailing your answer sheet(s) to Western Schools, we recommend you make a copy as a backup.*

ABOUT THIS COURSE

A "Pretest" is provided with each course to test your current knowledge base regarding the subject matter contained within this course. Your "Final Exam" is a multiple choice examination. **You will find the exam questions at the end of each chapter.** Some smaller hour courses include the exam at the end of the book.

In the event the course has less than 100 questions, leave the remaining answer boxes on the FasTrax answer sheet blank. **Use a __black pen__ to fill in your answer sheet.**

A PASSING SCORE

You must score 70% or better in order to pass this course and receive your Certificate of Completion. Should you fail to achieve the required score, we will send you an additional FasTrax answer sheet so that you may make a second attempt to pass the course. Western Schools will allow you three chances to pass the same course…*at no extra charge!* After three failed attempts to pass the same course, your file will be closed.

RECORDING YOUR HOURS

Please monitor the time it takes to complete this course using the handy log sheet on the other side of this page. See below for transferring study hours to the course evaluation.

COURSE EVALUATIONS

In this course book you will find a short evaluation about the course you are soon to complete. This information is vital to providing the school with feedback on this course. The course evaluation answer section is in the lower right hand corner of the FasTrax answer sheet marked "Evaluation" with answers marked 1–25. Your answers are important to us, please take five minutes to complete the evaluation.

On the back of the FasTrax instruction sheet there is additional space to make any comments about the course, the school, and suggested new curriculum. Please mail the FasTrax instruction sheet, with your comments, back to Western Schools in the envelope provided with your course order.

TRANSFERRING STUDY TIME

Upon completion of the course, transfer the total study time from your log sheet to question #25 in the Course Evaluation. The answers will be in ranges, please choose the proper hour range that best represents your study time. You MUST log your study time under question #25 on the course evaluation.

EXTENSIONS

You have 2 years from the date of enrollment to complete this course. A six (6) month extension may be purchased. If after 30 months from the original enrollment date you do not complete the course, *your file will be closed and no certificate can be issued.*

CHANGE OF ADDRESS?

In the event you have moved during the completion of this course please call our student services department at 1-800-618-1670 and we will update your file.

A GUARANTEE YOU'LL GIVE HIGH HONORS TO

If any continuing education course fails to meet your expectations or if you are not satisfied in any manner, for any reason, you may return it for an exchange or a refund (less shipping and handling) within 30 days. Software, video and audio courses must be returned unopened.

Thank you for enrolling at Western Schools!

WESTERN SCHOOLS
P.O. Box 1930
Brockton, MA 02303
(800) 438-8888
www.westernschools.com

Diabetes Nursing Care:
Overview and Management

WESTERN SCHOOLS

21 Bristol Drive

South Easton, MA 02375

Please use this log to total the number of hours you spend reading the text and taking the final examination (use 50-min hours).

Date	Hours Spent
_____	_____
_____	_____
_____	_____
_____	_____
_____	_____
_____	_____
_____	_____
_____	_____
_____	_____
_____	_____
_____	_____
_____	_____
_____	_____
_____	_____

TOTAL [   ]

Please log your study hours with submission of your final exam. To log your study time, fill in the appropriate circle under question 25 of the FasTrax® answer sheet under the "Evaluation" section.

PLEASE LOG YOUR STUDY HOURS WITH SUBMISSION OF YOUR FINAL EXAM. Please choose which best represents the total study hours it took to complete this 30 hour course.

A. less than 25 hours

B. 25–28 hours

C. 29–32 hours

D. greater than 32 hours

Diabetes Nursing Care:
Overview and Management

WESTERN SCHOOLS' NURSING
CONTINUING EDUCATION EVALUATION

Instructions: Mark your answers to the following questions with a black pen on the "Evaluation" section of your FasTrax® answer sheet provided with this course. You should not return this sheet. Please use the scale below to rate the following statements:

A   Agree Strongly   C   Disagree Somewhat
B   Agree Somewhat   D   Disagree Strongly

The course content met the following educational objectives:

1. Described the metabolic changes and resulting symptoms which occur in the chronic condition of Diabetes Mellitus.

2. Discussed the role of nutrition and diet in the overall management of Diabetes Mellitus.

3. Described the benefits of and the guidelines for exercise in the person with diabetes.

4. Discussed uses of and mechanism of action for the current medications used as therapy for diabetes.

5. Discussed the various types of monitoring done in diabetes management.

6. Identified the special issues involved in the management of patients with diabetes such as aging, surgery and traveling.

7. Identified signs and symptoms of acute complications of diabetes.

8. Discussed signs, symptoms, and treatments of the long-term microvascular and macrovascular complications of diabetes.

9. Discussed how support systems, stress, and other psychosocial factors impacted the diabetic patient and family.

10. Discussed areas of research being pursued in the field of diabetes.

11. Discussed utilizing the nursing process in caring for the patient with Diabetes Mellitus.

12. The content of this course was relevant to the objectives.

13. This offering met my professional educational needs.

14. The objectives met the overall purpose/goal of the course.

15. The course was generally well written and the subject matter explained thoroughly. (If no please explain on the back of the FasTrax instruction sheet.)

16. The content of this course was appropriate for home study.

17. The final examination was well written and at an appropriate level for the content of the course.

Please complete the following research questions in order to help us better meet your educational needs. Pick the ONE answer which is most appropriate.

18. For your LAST renewal did you take more Continuing Education contact hours than required by your state, if so, how many?

    A. 1–15 hours

    B. 16–30 hours

    C. 31 or more hours

    D. No, I only take the state required minimum

19. Do you usually exceed the contact hours required for your state license renewal, if so, why?

    A. Yes, I have more than one state license

    B. Yes, to meet additional special association Continuing Education requirements

    C. Yes, for professional self-interest/cross-training

    D. No, I only take the state required minimum

20. What nursing shift do you most commonly work?

    A. Morning Shift (Any shift starting after 3:00am or before 11:00am)

    B. Day/Afternoon Shift (Any shift starting after 11:00am or before 7:00pm)

    C. Night Shift (Any shift starting after 7:00pm or before 3:00am)

    D. I work rotating shifts

21. What was the SINGLE most important reason you chose this course?

    A. Low Price

    B. New or Newly revised course

    C. High interest/Required course topic

    D. Number of Contact Hours Needed

22. Where do you work? (If your place of employment is not listed below, please leave this question blank.)

    A. Hospital

    B. Medical Clinic/Group Practice/ HMO/office setting

    C. Long Term Care/Rehabilitation Facility/Nursing Home

    D. Home Health Care Agency

23. Which field do you specialize in?

    A. Medical/Surgical

    B. Geriatrics

    C. Pediatrics/Neonatal

    D. Other

24. For your last renewal, how many months BEFORE your license expiration date did you order your course materials?

    A. 1–3 months

    B. 4–6 months

    C. 7–12 months

    D. Greater than 12 months

25. **PLEASE LOG YOUR STUDY HOURS WITH SUBMISSION OF YOUR FINAL EXAM.** Please choose which best represents the total study hours it took to complete this 30 hour course.

    A. less than 25 hours

    B. 25–28 hours

    C. 29–32 hours

    D. greater than 32 hours

CONTENTS

PRETEST

Begin by taking the pretest. Compare your answers on the pretest to the answer key (located in the back of the book). Circle those test items that you missed. The pretest answer key indicates the course chapters where the content of that question is discussed. Circle the answers to the pretest questions. Do not log pretest questions on the Faxtrax answer sheet.

Next, read each chapter. Focus special attention on the chapters where you made incorrect answer choices. Exam questions are provided at the end of each chapter so that you can assess your progress and understanding of the material.

1. Non-insulin-dependent Diabetes Mellitus (type 2) is associated with which of the following?

   a. Tendency to ketosis
   b. Deficiency in insulin
   c. Obesity
   d. Antibodies to islet cells

2. Two months after diagnosis of type 1 diabetes, a patient who has normal blood glucose levels and requires less insulin than before is probably experiencing which of the following?

   a. Somogyi phenomenon
   b. Dawn phenomenon
   c. Caliph's syndrome
   d. Honeymoon period

3. What is the cause of polyuria in diabetes?

   a. A high renal threshold
   b. Osmotic diuresis
   c. Increased thirst
   d. Dehydration

4. Which of the following statements about type 2 diabetes is correct?

   a. It is the most frequently occurring diabetes.
   b. It usually occurs in children and young adults.
   c. It is typified by people who are thin at the time of diagnosis.
   d. It starts abruptly with clearly defined signs and symptoms.

5. Which of the following is a food containing 15 grams of carbohydrate that can be used on a sick day by a patient who has diabetes?

   a. One-half cup of ice cream
   b. Eight soda crackers
   c. One cup of orange juice
   d. One-half cup of cream soup

6. In the carbohydrate counting system for patients with diabetes, which of the following food groups is counted as 15 grams of carbohydrate?

   a. Fats
   b. Meats
   c. Milk
   d. Fruits

7. To lose 1 pound (0.45 kg) of body weight per week, a person must reduce his or her daily caloric requirement by how many calories?

    a. 1000

    b. 200

    c. 500

    d. 250

8. Which of the following statements about exercise and diabetes is correct?

    a. Aerobic exercise is too strenuous for a patient with diabetes.

    b. Exercise activities should be limited to brisk walking.

    c. Exercise increases the risk of diabetic complications in all patients.

    d. Aerobic exercise is generally recommended for patients with diabetes.

9. An example of aerobic exercise is

    a. brisk walking.

    b. weight lifting.

    c. sprinting.

    d. body building.

10. What is the best site for injection of insulin for a patient who is planning to exercise by swimming laps?

    a. Leg

    b. Arm

    c. Thigh

    d. Abdomen

11. Oral antidiabetes agents are usually used to treat which type of diabetes?

    a. Gestational

    b. Juvenile

    c. Type 1

    d. Type 2

12. Which oral antidiabetes agent is most likely to cause flushing, nausea, and vomiting when alcohol is ingested?

    a. Chlorpropamide

    b. Glipizide

    c. Glyburide

    d. Tolbutamide

13. Which oral antidiabetes agent has an effect on the liver?

    a. Acetohexamide (Dymelor®)

    b. Glipizide (Glucotrol®)

    c. Metformin (Glucophage®)

    d. Tolbutamide (Orinase®)

14. Which of the following patients with diabetes must self-monitor blood glucose levels?

    a. Patients with altered renal thresholds

    b. Patients who use insulin infusion pumps

    c. Patients who have type 2 diabetes

    d. Patients with impaired fasting glucose

15. According to the standards established by the American Diabetes Association, the level of diabetes control for a patient with average fasting blood glucose levels of 225 mg/dl is considered which of the following?

    a. Normal

    b. Acceptable

    c. High normal

    d. Poor

16. In a patient with a renal threshold of 200 mg/dl, what does a 7 a.m. urine test that is positive for glucose indicate about the patient's concentration of blood glucose?

   a. It has been greater than 200 mg/dl since the last voiding.

   b. It may be less than 200 mg/dl now but has been more than 200 mg/dl sometime since the last voiding.

   c. It is greater than 200 mg/dl at 7 a.m.

   d. It has not been less than 200 mg/dl since the last voiding.

17. Which of the following statements about insulin requirements for patients with type 1 diabetes who are undergoing major surgery is correct?

   a. They usually require less insulin than usual.

   b. They do not require insulin on the day of surgery.

   c. They often require increased amounts of insulin.

   d. They usually require no changes in their insulin dosages.

18. An important goal in the care of a 2-year-old with diabetes is to do which of the following?

   a. Encourage the child to help with glucose testing.

   b. Avoid hypoglycemia.

   c. Promote the Mauriac system.

   d. Test for ketones twice a day.

19. How does hyperglycemia impede infection healing in a diabetic foot?

   a. By worsening sensory neuropathy

   b. By interfering with leukocyte function

   c. By decreasing circulation

   d. By inducing swelling

20. Which of the following is one of the most common fungal infections in females with diabetes?

   a. Vulvovaginitis

   b. Folliculitis

   c. Necrobiosis lipoidica diabeticorum

   d. Carbuncles

21. Which of the following is an early sign of diabetic renal disease?

   a. Azotemia

   b. Albuminuria

   c. Nocturia

   d. Creatinuria

22. Which of the following statements about distal symmetric polyneuropathy is correct?

   a. It is the least common form of neuropathy.

   b. The signs and symptoms develop unpredictably.

   c. It is characterized by sensory changes that begin in the fingers and toes.

   d. It always causes intense and "shooting" pain in the calf.

23. What percentage of patients with diabetes probably do not adhere to their diabetes management plan?

   a. 90

   b. 75

   c. 50

   d. 10

24. Successful management of diabetes is directly and mainly dependent on which of the following?

   a. Hereditary predisposition to atherosclerosis

   b. The patient's acceptance of the condition

   c. Correct timing of insulin injections

   d. Dietary therapy that restricts simple carbohydrates

25. In evaluating the use of glucagon for a patient who has severe hypoglycemia, the nurse knows which of the following about glucagon?

    a. It may have to be given several times until the person responds.

    b. It should be used only in hospitalized patients and given via an intravenous line.

    c. It is effective only if hepatic glycogen is available.

    d. It is the treatment of choice for mild hypoglycemia.

PREFACE

Diabetes Mellitus is a chronic metabolic disease that is becoming more prevalent. With this increase comes the need for well-qualified nurses to care for and teach patients who have diabetes.

In the past few years, major breakthroughs in diabetes research and methods of care have opened new doors to better management of this disorder. The immediate dangers associated with both extremely high and extremely low blood glucose levels have long been recognized. Recently, it has become possible to detect a direct relationship between the long-term elevation of blood glucose levels and some of the most serious complications of diabetes: strokes, heart attacks, blindness, loss of limbs, and renal disease.

Until a cure or prevention is found, there is a need for caregivers who are knowledgeable about diabetes and its management. This book is intended to help maximize nurses' skills and knowledge by providing the latest and most current information on diabetes. Throughout, the emphasis is on educating patients about self-care in the four major techniques of diabetes management: diet, exercise, medication, and home blood glucose monitoring.

The information contained in this text is applicable to a wide variety of patient care settings. By facilitating optimal diabetes care, the knowledge gained by studying this material will enhance and enrich the experiences of both patients and nurses.

CHAPTER 1

PATHOPHYSIOLOGY OF DIABETES

CHAPTER OBJECTIVE

After studying this chapter, the reader will be able to describe the metabolic changes and resulting signs and symptoms that occur in chronic Diabetes Mellitus.

LEARNING OBJECTIVES

After completing this chapter, the reader will be able to:

1. Specify the distinguishing characteristics of type 1 and type 2 diabetes.

2. Indicate known and suspected factors in the etiology of diabetes.

3. Specify epidemiologic features of diabetes.

4. Recognize signs and symptoms of diabetes.

5. List the definitions of physiologic processes important in glucose metabolism.

6. Recognize the effects of hormones important in the regulation of glucose metabolism.

INTRODUCTION

The term Diabetes Mellitus means the running through of sugar. Diabetes has been known since the first century A.D. when Aretaeus of Cappadocia described the disorder as a chronic affliction that resulted in intense thirst and voluminous amounts of honey-sweet urine: "the melting down of flesh into urine" (Waif, 1980). On the basis of these signs and symptoms, the Greeks and the Romans gave diabetes its name:

DIABETES = SIPHON (frequent urination)

MELLITUS = HONEY (sugar in the urine)

Currently, diabetes affects approximately 16 million Americans. For the last ten year period, diabetes increased 9% annually, and it is estimated that for every person known to have diabetes, there is one unknown who has minimal signs and symptoms. Each year diabetes is diagnosed in an additional 600,000 Americans. If this trend continues, the number of people with diabetes in the United States will double every 15 years. The overall prevalence rate for diabetes in the United States is about 6%. However specific subgroups have a much higher prevalence of the disease than the population as a whole (American Diabetes Association, 1999). As long as more and more people become overweight, become less physically active and as life expectancy lengthens, the incidence of diabetes will continue to increase.

The discovery of insulin by two Canadians, Banting and Best, in 1921 transformed the once-fatal disease of type 1 diabetes into a chronic health problem. Before that time, early death of young children and adults through virtual starvation and tremendous suffering was almost always the eventual outcome of diabetes.

Diabetes continues to extract a tremendous toll:

1

- Diabetes with its related complications is the sixth leading cause of death.

- Diabetes accounts for 5–6% of hospital admissions.

- Nearly 25% of all new dialysis patients have diabetes.

- People with diabetes are two to four times more likely than those without the disorder to die of heart disease and two to six times more likely to have a stroke.

- Diabetic eye disease is the No. 1 cause of new blindness.

- Diabetes is the major cause of nontraumatic amputations.

Direct and indirect costs for diabetes are nearly $92 billion annually and account for nearly 11% of total health care costs in the United States (ADA, 1999).

Two long term, recently concluded studies; the Diabetes Control and Complications Trial and the United Kingdom Prospective Study (see Chapter 11 for discussion) have shown that improved blood sugars can reduce the complications associated with diabetes. Thus there is a definite movement on the part of diabetes professionals to promote early diagnosis and effective treatment of diabetes.

PHYSIOLOGY OF GLUCOSE METABOLISM

All bodily activities require energy. Metabolism is the process through which carbohydrates, proteins, and fats from food are converted into energy for use by cells. Glucose is the major fuel source of the body. Although many tissues and organ systems can use other sources such as fatty acids and ketones for fuel, the brain and nervous system rely almost exclusively on glucose as a fuel source. The nervous system cannot store or synthesize glucose to meet its energy needs. In the fed and early fasting state, the nervous system requires about 100–115g of glucose to meet its daily metabolic needs (Davidson, J., 1986). Without a source of glucose, a person cannot live.

Glucose is obtained from the metabolism of a variety of dietary sources: table sugar; milk sugar (lactose); fruit sugar (fructose); and complex sugars of vegetables, breads, and starches. In addition, 60% of the protein and 10% of the fat in the diet contribute glucose (Lodewick, 1988).

The glucose ingested in the diet is transported from the gastrointestinal tract through the portal vein to the liver before going into the circulatory system for use by the cells. Excess glucose is converted to fatty acids and stored in fat cells as triglycerides or is converted to glycogen and stored in the liver and skeletal muscle *(Figure 1-1)*. Because the liver both stores and synthesizes glucose, it acts as a buffer system to regulate blood levels of the sugar. Through the body's homeostatic mechanism, if blood glucose levels are high, glucose is stored in the liver as glycogen. If blood glucose levels are low, the liver releases stored glucose.

Glucose is transported through the bloodstream to the cells where insulin binds with the receptor sites on the surface of target cells (cells that require insulin for glucose metabolism). This binding makes the wall of the cell permeable and allows the glucose to enter *(Figure 1-2)*.

Metabolic Processes

Three metabolic processes are important in ensuring a supply of glucose for body fuel. Glycolysis is the process through which glucose is broken down into water and carbon dioxide with the release of energy. Glycogenolysis is the breakdown of stored glycogen (from the liver or skeletal muscles). This process is controlled by the action of two hormones: epinephrine and glucagon. Epinephrine is primarily effective in breaking

FIGURE 1-1 Glucose Metabolism

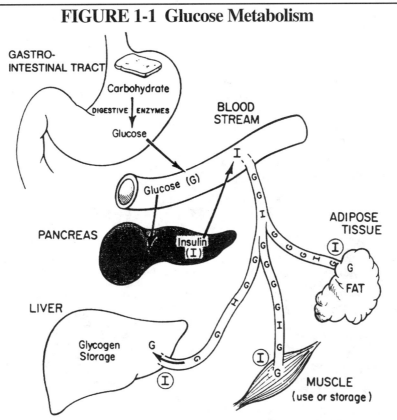

Carbohydrate is the primary source of energy for the body. The body gets its carbohydrate fuel from sugars and starches. These are digested in the gastrointestinal tract into simple sugars (e.g., glucose), which pass into the bloodstream. Glucose in the bloodstream stimulates the pancreas to secrete insulin. Insulin directs the glucose to muscle for use or storage, to liver for storage as glycogen, or to adipose tissue for storage of fat.

Source: Krall, L., & Beaser, R. (1989). *Joslin diabetes manual* (p. 9). Philadelphia: Lea & Febiger.

down glycogen in the muscle, whereas glucagon is primarily effective in breaking down glycogen in the liver. Glucose released from the liver can be directly released to the bloodstream and used by the nervous system.

Gluconeogenesis is the building of glucose from new sources. Amino acids, lactate, and glycerol can be converted into glucose. Several hormones stimulate gluconeogenesis, including glucagon, glucocorticoid hormones, and thyroid hormones. Most of the gluconeogenesis occurs in the liver. Although fatty acids can be used directly as fuel by many body cells, they cannot be converted to glucose.

Hormonal Control Of Metabolism

Several hormones are important in the regulation of glucose metabolism.

Insulin

Insulin is secreted by a small group of cells called beta cells in the islets of Langerhans in the pancreas. Surprisingly, the beta cells account for less than 1% of the total cells of the pancreas. The insulin molecule consists of two polypeptide chains with a connecting C peptide link. Therefore, the amount of insulin a person is secreting can be determined by measuring levels of C peptide. Once insulin is secreted into the general circulation, its half-life is about 15 min.

Insulin is the only hormone known to have the direct effect of decreasing the level of glucose in the blood. It decreases the level by promoting transport of glucose into skeletal muscle and adipose tissue. Insulin also decreases the breakdown of glucose and fat stores and stimulates synthesis of both glycogen and triglyceride. It also promotes

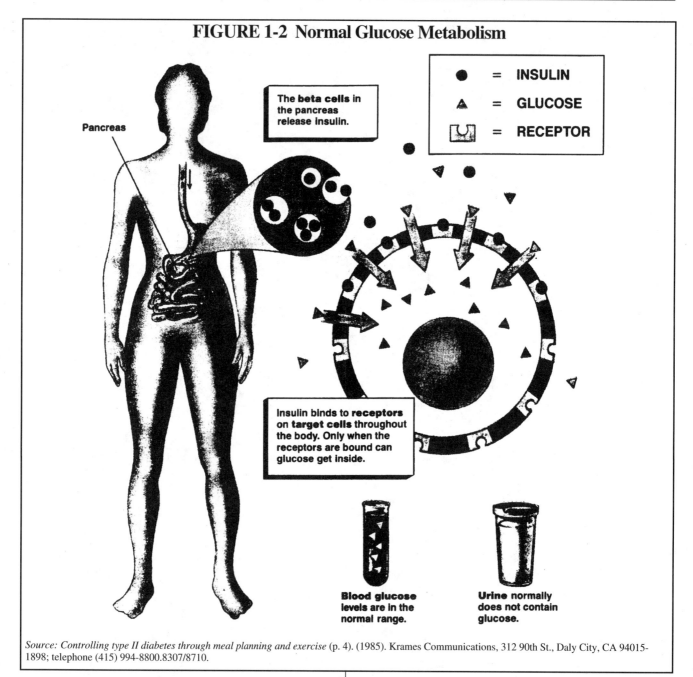

FIGURE 1-2 Normal Glucose Metabolism

Pancreas

The **beta cells** in the pancreas release insulin.

● = **INSULIN**

▲ = **GLUCOSE**

⊔ = **RECEPTOR**

Insulin binds to **receptors** on **target cells** throughout the body. Only when the receptors are bound can glucose get inside.

Blood glucose levels are in the normal range.

Urine normally does not contain glucose.

Source: Controlling type II diabetes through meal planning and exercise (p. 4). (1985). Krames Communications, 312 90th St., Daly City, CA 94015-1898; telephone (415) 994-8800.8307/8710.

transport of amino acids into body cells and accelerates protein synthesis in the cell.

Secretion of insulin is regulated through blood glucose levels, increasing when blood levels of glucose increase and decreasing when glucose is lowered in the blood stream. Insulin is released in two phases. The first phase occurs within the first 10 minutes after the ingestion of glucose. This is the insulin that was stored in the beta cells. The second phase is the release of newly synthesized insulin. Insulin levels rise within minutes after a meal, peak at about 30 minutes, and fall back to baseline within 3 hours.

Insulin is essential for the glucose supply of most cells that constitute a large percentage of body mass and energy expenditure and perform a large part of tissue building and repair. Not all tissues depend on insulin for glucose to enter the cells. These insulin-independent tissues that allow glucose to enter freely are often the site of complications associated with diabetes (eyes, erythrocytes, kidneys, and nerves). The brain is also an insulin-independent tissue.

Amylin

A second beta cell hormone, amylin, was recently discovered. The effects of amylin appear to be twofold:

1. Amylin in conjunction with insulin suppresses the secretion of glucagon by the liver which should reduce the production of hepatic glucose postprandially and

2. Amylin slows the transfer of nutrients to the intestine, thus slowing the appearance of glucose from meals into the bloodstream (Amylin, 1998).

Glucagon

Glucagon is produced in the alpha cells of the islets of Langerhans in the pancreas. It also is transported via the portal vein to the liver, where it exerts its action. Glucagon acts in opposition to insulin. It stimulates the breakdown of glycogen and fats to glucose and promotes gluconeogenesis from fats and proteins to increase glucose levels.

Catecholamines

The catecholamines, epinephrine and norepinephrine, help maintain blood glucose levels during stress by: (1) inhibiting insulin release and decreasing movement of glucose into cells; (2) promoting glycogenolysis by converting muscle and liver glycogen to glucose; and (3) increasing lipase activity, which causes mobilization of fatty acids and thereby conserves glucose. The conservation of blood glucose mediated by these actions is important in the homeostatic effect, which occurs in hypoglycemia to increase the level of blood glucose.

Somatostatin

Somatostatin is produced in the pancreas by the delta cells in the Islets of Langerhans. This hormone inhibits the secretion of insulin, glucagon, and growth hormone. The complete physiologic action and importance of somatostatin are not yet fully known.

Growth Hormones

An increase in the serum level of growth hormones generally causes an increase in blood glucose levels by decreasing peripheral utilization of glucose. This increase in blood glucose levels stimulates beta cells to produce increasing amounts of insulin. In people with higher than normal levels of growth hormone (e.g., acromegaly), the stimulation can cause the beta cells to literally "burn out," and diabetes develops.

Glucocorticoid Hormones

Cortisol and other glucocorticoid hormones stimulate gluconeogenesis in the liver. The rate of glucose production is increased dramatically, as much as 6- to 10-fold. Prolonged elevation of the adrenal corticoid hormones in persons predisposed to diabetes can lead to hyperglycemia and the development of Diabetes Mellitus.

PATHOPHYSIOLOGY OF DIABETES

Diabetes is a chronic state of high blood sugars which result from the combination of persistent elevations in fasting blood glucose and excessive postprandial hyperglycemia. Both of these abnormalities increase the 24 hour concentrations of blood glucose, elevation of the hemoglobin A1c (see chapter 5) and an increased risk for the development of long term complications. Diabetes can be due to insulin deficiency or a number of other metabolic defects.

DIAGNOSIS OF DIABETES

The diagnostic, screening and classification of diabetes is established by the Expert Committee of the American Diabetes

---

TABLE 1-1
Diagnostic Criteria for Diabetes Mellitus

NONPREGNANT ADULTS

Criteria for Diabetes Mellitus.** Diagnosis of Diabetes Mellitus in nonpregnant adults is made in those who have one of the following:

- casual plasma glucose level of ≥200 mg/dl plus the classic signs and symptoms of diabetes (e.g,. polyuria, polydipsia, polyphagia and unexplained weight loss)

- fasting plasma glucose level of ≥126 mg/dl

- 2 hour plasma glucose level of ≥200 mg/dl during an oral glucose tolerance test

** In the absence of unequivocal hyperglycemia with metabolic decompensation, these criteria should be confirmed by repeat testing on a different day.

Criteria for Impaired Glucose Tolerance. A diagnosis of impaired glucose tolerance (IGT) is made when an individual has:

- fasting plasma glucose level of ≥110 mg/dl but <126 mg/dl

Criteria for Impaired Fasting Glucose. A diagnosis of impaired fasting glucose (IFG) is made when an individual has:

- fasting plasma glucose level of ≥110 mg/dl but <140 mg/dl

PREGNANT WOMEN

Criteria for Gestational Diabetes. Screening for gestational diabetes is recommended for women over 25 years of age and for women less than age 25 with increased risk factors such as: obesity, first degree relatives with diabetes and women who are Hispanic, Native American or African American.

- After an oral glucose load of 100 gm, diagnosis of gestational diabetes may be made if two plasma glucose values equal or exceed the following:

Fasting	1hr	2 hr	3 hr
105	190	165	145

Association (ADA , 1999). The criteria for the diagnosis *(Table 1-1)* of diabetes are:

1. Symptoms of diabetes (e.g., polyuria, polydipsia, weight loss) plus a casual (without regard to time of day or time since last meal) plasma glucose concentration equal to or greater than 200 mg/dl.

or

2. Fasting (no caloric intake for 8 or more hours) plasma glucose equal to or greater than 126 mg/dl.

or

3. A two hour plasma glucose equal to or greater than 200 mg/dl on a OGTT (oral glucose tolerance test of 75 g glucose load).

The diagnosis of diabetes is an important one, so a diagnosis is made only when any of the three tests above is repeated on a different day and yields the same results.

Different criteria are defined for children and pregnant women (Chapter 6). The diagnosis of impaired glucose tolerance is used for people who have abnormal plasma glucose levels that do not meet the criteria for diabetes.

In addition two categories of impaired glucose functioning are defined:

1. Impaired Fasting Glucose (IFG) is diagnosed when fasting glucose levels are greater than 110 mg/dl but less than 126 mg/dl. This is a metabolic state of impaired glucose homeostasis between normal and Diabetes Mellitus. IFG is not a category of Diabetes Mellitus.

2. Impaired Glucose Tolerance (IGT) is diagnosed when the 2 hour OGTT values are greater than 140 mg/dl but less than 200 mg/dl. This is also an impaired state of glucose homeostasis between normal and diabetes and is not a category of Diabetes Mellitus.

CLASSIFICATION OF DIABETES

Diabetes has been classified *(Table 1-2)* by the National Diabetes Data Group and the World Health Organization and has been recently updated by the ADA (1999).

Type 1

Type 1 diabetes *(Figure 1-3)* formerly known as insulin dependent diabetes (IDDM) affects approximately 700,000 individuals in this country. It can develop at any age, although most cases are generally diagnosed when the patient is less than 30 years old. Previously, this type of diabetes was often referred to as "juvenile diabetes," because its onset often occurs in childhood. Type 1 diabetes usually appears suddenly and progresses quickly. Patients usually seek medical care within days to 2 or 3 weeks because of the severity of the signs and symptoms.

Because patients with type 1 diabetes are insulinopenic (little or no production of insulin), insulin therapy is essential to prevent ketoacidosis and death. These patients are usually lean and often have had marked recent weight loss, polyuria, polyphagia, and polydipsia before diagnosis. They often have antibodies to islet cells (ICA) and a diminished level of C peptide at the time of diagnosis.

Immunologic Factors in Type 1 Diabetes

It is believed that the immune system attacks and destroys the insulin producing beta cells in the pancreas. The actual disease process begins as long as nine years before the onset of clinical symptoms. Hyperglycemia and symptoms consistent with the diagnosis of diabetes develop only after more than 90% of the secretory capacity of the beta cell mass has been destroyed. There is a genetic propensity of type 1 diabetes. The risk of developing type 1 diabetes in the general population ranges from 0.1–0.25%. The risk is increased in children of parents with diabetes to a range of 2–5%.

A "trigger" is necessary for the development of the disease in those with the genetic propensity.

Several possible triggers for the development of this autoimmune process have been investigated, including viruses (the number of cases diagnosed increases in the flu and cold season), environmental toxins, serum, and drugs.

Individuals with type 1 diabetes are also prone to other autoimmune disorders, particularly the thyroid disorders of Graves disease and Hashimoto thyroiditis, Addison's Disease, vitiligo and pernicious anemia.

FIGURE 1-3 Type 1 Diabetes

People with type 1 diabetes have enough receptors, but they can't produce enough insulin.

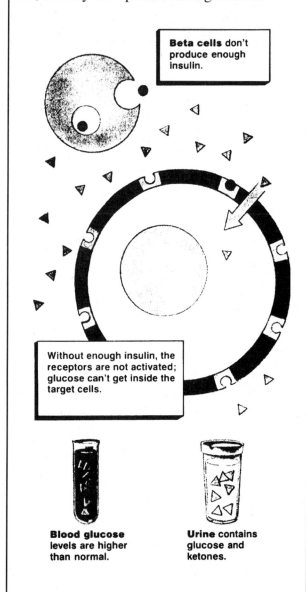

Beta cells don't produce enough insulin.

Without enough insulin, the receptors are not activated; glucose can't get inside the target cells.

Blood glucose levels are higher than normal.

Urine contains glucose and ketones.

Less Insulin

Receptor sites are plentiful, but the beta cells can't secrete enough insulin to bind to them. Because the target cells can't take in glucose, blood sugar levels rise. The body switches to using fat for energy producing harmful byproducts called ketones. As with type 2 diabetes, extra glucose spills over into the urine.

Source: Controlling type II diabetes through meal planning and exercise (p. 5). (1985). Krames Communications, 312 90th St., Daly City, CA 94015-1898; telephone (415) 994-8800.8307/8710.

Signs and Symptoms

The signs and symptoms of type 1 diabetes are usually acute *(Table 1-3)* and have a rapid onset, causing the patient to seek medical care because of a feeling that something is terribly wrong.

The classic signs and symptoms of diabetes are the three "polys": polyuria (excessive urination), polydipsia (excessive thirst), and polyphagia (excessive hunger). These three are related to the elevated levels of blood glucose (hyperglycemia) and the "spilling" of glucose into the urine (glycosuria).

When the body cannot properly metabolize glucose, hyperglycemia occurs. The normal renal threshold (the amount of glucose filtered by the glomeruli of the kidney) is 180 mg/dl (9.9 mmol/L). If the blood level of glucose is sufficiently high, this threshold is exceeded, and glucose spills into the urine. Because of the osmotic diuresis that occurs with glycosuria, a large loss of water and polyuria occur. Thirst is due to the intracellular dehydration that occurs, and patients often have polydipsia, including consumption of literally gallons of fluids per day. Dramatic weight loss in a short time (*ex:* 10–20 pounds in a 2 week period) despite polyphagia and markedly increased food intake is common in patients with type 1 diabetes. The reasons for weight loss are (1) osmotic diuresis with loss of body fluids (dehydration), (2) loss of fluid through vomiting, and (3) loss of body tissue because the body is forced to use its fat stores and cellular proteins as fuel sources because of a lack of insulin. Dryness of the mouth is another symptom that occurs because of the cellular dehydration.

Nausea, vomiting, a "fruity" breath odor, and Kussmaul's breathing are all indications of ketoacidosis, which is due to the use of body stores to produce energy (type 1 diabetes). These are dangerous signs and symptoms and warrant immediate medical attention.

Profound fatigue and lack of energy are often complaints that cause a person with diabetes to seek care. They are due to lack of proper cellular nutrition, because the glucose normally used for energy is not available.

Blurring of vision is another common and distressing symptom. It is due to swelling in the lens of the eye associated with hyperglycemia and is reversible with control of glucose levels.

Honeymoon Phase (Remission)

At the time of diagnosis of type 1 diabetes in patients with symptomatic hyperglycemia or ketoacidosis, the remaining functioning beta cells are heavily stressed. Somewhat later, when insulin injections have allowed these cells to recover, the cells may be able to secrete sufficient insulin to allow the patient to dramatically reduce or even discontinue insulin injections for a time. This period is referred to as the "honeymoon," because it is only temporary. Eventually, all function of the beta cells will be lost. The honeymoon lasts a short time, usually a matter of weeks to months. Rarely, it lasts for more than a year before insulin is again needed.

Type 2

Type 2 diabetes *(Figure 1-4)*, formerly called non insulin dependent diabetes (NIDDM) or type II diabetes, are neither insulin dependent nor ketosis prone. However, insulin by injection may be necessary to achieve the desired control of blood glucose levels and to correct persistent hyperglycemia. Typically, patients with type 2 diabetes have insulin resistance in the form of decreased tissue sensitivity or decreased responsiveness to insulin. The resistance may be due to the reduction of insulin binding to its receptors in peripheral tissues, a reduction in the number of receptors, alteration of intracellular function (e.g., postreceptor defect), or a combination of these. In addition, patients may have abnormalities of hepatic glucose production. Higher than normal amounts of glucose are released from the liver before food intake,

---

TABLE 1-2
Types of Diabetes Mellitus and Other Categories of Glucose Intolerance

CLINICAL CLASSES	DISTINGUISHING CHARACTERISTICS
Type 1 Diabetes Mellitus	Patients may be of any age, are usually thin, and usually have abrupt onset of signs and symptoms with insulinopenia before the age of 30. These patients have hyperglycemia, positive urine ketone tests, often experience profound weight loss, polyuria, polydipsia, polyphagia, and polydipsia. They are dependent on insulin therapy to prevent ketoacidosis and sustain life.
Type 2 Diabetes Mellitus	Patients are usually older than 30 years at diagnosis, obese, and have relatively few classic symptoms. Diagnosis is often made in conjunction with a routine physical exam or another health care problem. They are not prone to ketoacidosis except during periods of stress. Although not dependent on exogenous insulin for survival, they may require it for adequate control of hyperglycemia.
Other specific types of Diabetes Mellitus	Patients with other types of Diabetes Mellitus have certain associated conditions or syndromes.
Impaired glucose tolerance	Patients with impaired glucose tolerance have plasma glucose levels that are higher than normal but not diagnostic for Diabetes Mellitus.
Gestational Diabetes Mellitus	Patients with gestational Diabetes Mellitus have onset or discovery of glucose intolerance during pregnancy.

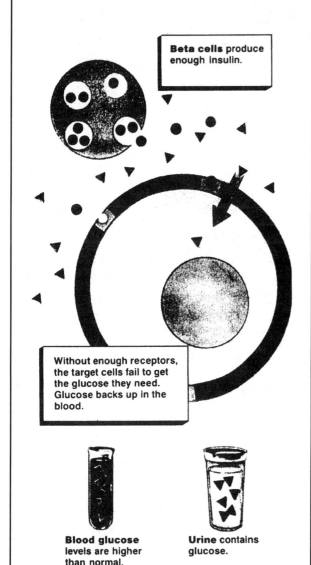

FIGURE 1-4 Type 2 Diabetes

Most people with type 2 diabetes have more than enough insulin, but not enough receptors.

Beta cells produce enough insulin.

Without enough receptors, the target cells fail to get the glucose they need. Glucose backs up in the blood.

Blood glucose levels are higher than normal.

Urine contains glucose.

Fewer Insulin Receptors

Obesity often associated with lack of exercise, reduces the number of insulin receptor sites. Then, because the target cells can't take in glucose, blood sugar levels rise. The kidneys are unable to reabsorb all the glucose from the blood they filter, so some will pass into the urine.

Source: Controlling type II diabetes through meal planning and exercise (p. 5). (1985). Krames Communications, 312 90th St., Daly City, CA 94015-1898; telephone (415) 994-8800.8307/8710.

and the level of glucose uptake after food is eaten is lower than normal. Patients with type 2 diabetes are not prone to ketoacidosis because enough insulin is present to prevent excess fat breakdown to supply energy.

These patients may have insulin levels that appear normal or are elevated. However insulin secretion is defective and insufficient to compensate for the insulin resistance. Insulin resistance may improve with weight reduction, increased physical activity or medication.

Although this type of diabetes can occur at any age, it is most often diagnosed in a person after the age of 40 years. It has often been called "adult-onset diabetes" for this reason. Sixty to ninety percent of patients with type 2 diabetes are obese at the time of diagnosis or have a history of obesity, but the disorder can occur in the nonobese as well, especially in older persons.

Signs and Symptoms

Type 2 diabetes *(Table 1-3)* often goes undiagnosed for many years because of the gradual development of high blood glucose that is not severe enough for the person to notice any of the classic symptoms of diabetes. Type 2 diabetes is often diagnosed when a patient seeks medical care for another reason or may be discovered during a routine dental, eye or physical examination. It is estimated that a number of people may have had the disease for an average of 7–10 years at the time of diagnosis. Unfortunately by the time diagnosis is made, complications may have already developed.

Patients with type 2 diabetes may exhibit any of the symptoms of type 1 diabetes with a few exceptions. Weight loss is not characteristic of type 2 diabetes unless complications are occurring. Also as mentioned, these individuals do not exhibit ketoacidosis nor its symptoms of nausea and vomiting.

Symptoms that are more characteristic of type 2 diabetes include abnormalities of healing, commonly manifested as slow healing of sores, and an increased rate of occurrence of certain infections sometimes occur. Both hyperglycemia and glycosuria favor the growth of yeasts. Pruritus and vulvovaginitis due to candidal infections are common initial complaints in women. Men may seek medical care because of impotence or difficulties with sexual function. Tingling and numbness in the feet and hands are also common symptoms.

Syndrome X and Type 2 Diabetes

Syndrome X is the name of a group of metabolic factors and hypertension associated with type 2 diabetes that leads to cardiovascular disease. The components of Syndrome X include insulin resistance, hyperinsulinemia, hyperglycemia, decreased HDL cholesterol, increased triglycerides, elevated blood pressure and albuminuria. These factors are probably linked by insulin resistance and possibly a common genetic defect.

OTHER SPECIFIC TYPES OF DIABETES

Diabetes may also be due to or secondary to other conditions. These include pancreatic disease, diseases of excessive hormone production (*ex:* Cushing's syndrome, acromegaly, pheochromocytoma, primary aldosteronism, glucagonoma), diseases of the exocrine pancreas (*ex:* pancreatitis, cystic fibrosis, hemochromatosis), certain chemicals and medications (e.g., thiazide diuretics, psychoactive agents, glucocorticoids such as prednisone, catecholamines), and certain genetic syndromes (e.g., Turner's Syndrome, Huntington's chorea) (ADA, 1999).

Gestational Diabetes

The diagnosis of gestational Diabetes Mellitus is made when glucose intolerance has its onset or is first detected during pregnancy. After the pregnancy, if blood glucose levels return to normal, the

---

> ### TABLE 1-3
> ### The Warning Signs of Diabetes
>
> **Type 1 Diabetes Mellitus** (Symptoms develop rapidly)
> - Frequent urination (Frequent bed-wetting in children who have been toilet trained)
> - Excessive Thirst
> - Excessive Hunger
> - Weakness and fatigue
> - Drowsiness
> - Irritability
> - Blurred vision or any change in sight
> - Fruity breath
> - Nausea and vomiting
> - Sudden unexplained weight loss
>
> **Type 2 Diabetes Mellitus** (Symptoms usually develop gradually)
> - Any of the symptoms listed above (although usually not the last three listed above)
> - Tingling or numbness in legs, feet or fingers
> - Slow healing of cuts (esp on feet)
> - Frequent skin or vaginal infections or itchy skin

patient's diagnostic classification may be changed to previous abnormality of glucose tolerance. Women who have gestational Diabetes Mellitus have an increased risk for diabetes in the future.

Impaired Glucose Tolerance

The term impaired glucose tolerance is used when patients have glucose levels that are higher than normal but do not meet the criterion for a diagnosis of Diabetes Mellitus.

The National Diabetes Data Group recommends that the use of several terms be discouraged, including juvenile diabetes and adult-onset diabetes. The labels "borderline" and "chemical" diabetes are now redesignated as impaired glucose tolerance, and "prediabetes" has been replaced with either previous abnormality of glucose tolerance or potential abnormality of glucose tolerance.

EPIDEMIOLOGY AND RISK FACTORS

Approximately 80–90% of all cases of diabetes, diagnosed and undiagnosed, are thought to be type 2. Type 1 diabetes accounts for 5–10% of known cases. The remainder, or about 2%, is diabetes secondary to other conditions. Gestational Diabetes Mellitus occurs in 2–5% of pregnancies.

Lifestyle, genetics, and the environment are all risk factors for the development of diabetes. The incidence of type 1 diabetes is 1.5 times higher in whites than in blacks, with no difference for risk between males and females. The disorder will develop in 2–5% of the siblings of patients who have type 1 diabetes. Among identical twins, one of whom has type 1 diabetes the concordance rates are only 50%.

The most important risk factors for type 2 diabetes are obesity, sedentary lifestyle, increasing age (most cases occur in people 40 years and older), and family history. Studies indicate a 90–100% concordance for type 2 diabetes in identical twins. Rates are higher for blacks, Hispanics, and Native Americans than for whites. The Pima Indians of the Southwest have the highest prevalence of any group. In this group, the chance of diabetes developing is 50% after the age of 50 years. Type 2 diabetes occurs more frequently in women with prior history of gestational diabetes and in individuals with hypertension and dyslipidemia (ADA, 1999).

SCREENING FOR DIABETES

In order to identify as many cases of type 2 diabetes as early as possible and to prevent their complications, the ADA (1999) has established guidelines for screening patients. The guidelines advise that everyone over the age of 45 be tested for diabetes every three years. Individuals with additional risk factors should be tested earlier and more frequently. The risk factors for type 2 diabetes specified by the American Diabetes Association include:

- Obesity

- Having a close relative (parent, sibling, or child) with diabetes

- Being African-American, Latino, Native American or Asian

- Delivering a baby weighing more than 9 pounds or being diagnosed with gestational diabetes

- High blood pressure

- High density lipoprotein (HDL) at or below 35 mg/dl or a triglyceride level at or above 250 mg/dl

- Previously impaired glucose tolerance or impaired fasting glucose on testing

EXAM QUESTIONS

CHAPTER 1
Questions 1–9

1. Type 1 Diabetes Mellitus is associated with which of the following?

    a. Antibodies to islet cells

    b. Insulin resistance

    c. Postreceptor defects

    d. DR7 haplotype

2. Which of the following is characteristic of patients with type 2 diabetes?

    a. Ketosis

    b. Profound weight loss

    c. Obesity

    d. Low insulin levels

3. Etiologic factors for type 1 diabetes include

    a. obesity.

    b. excessive hepatic glucose production.

    c. an auto immune process.

    d. decreased number of receptor sites.

4. Gluconeogenesis is defined as which of the following?

    a. Breakdown of glucose into water and carbon dioxide with the release of energy

    b. Conversion of glucose to fatty acids

    c. Building of glucose from new sources

    d. Conversion of glycogen to glucose

5. What is the normal renal threshold, in milligrams per deciliter, for glucose in adults?

    a. 130

    b. 140

    c. 180

    d. 250

6. Which of the following is characteristic of uncontrolled type 1 Diabetes Mellitus?

    a. Dawn phenomenon

    b. Polyphagia with weight loss

    c. Honeymoon period

    d. Hypoglycemia

7. Syndrome X is associated with

    a. type 1 diabetes.

    b. children.

    c. type 2 diabetes.

    d. gestational diabetes.

8. A patient with type 2 diabetes will have which of the following laboratory results at the time of diagnosis?

    a. A fasting plasma glucose level higher than 126 mg/dl

    b. One of two plasma glucose levels greater than 250 mg/dl on an oral glucose tolerance test.

    c. A glycohemoglobin level higher than 12%.

    d. One postprandial plasma glucose level greater than 200 mg/dl and a fasting level less than 126 mg/dl on an oral glucose tolerance test.

9. What is the physiologic effect of the hormone glucagon?

    a. It stimulates the release of insulin from the pancreas.

    b. It helps insulin bind with the receptor sites on the cell.

    c. It stimulates the breakdown of glycogen to provide glucose.

    d. It decreases movement of glucose into the cells.

CHAPTER 2

NUTRITION AND DIETARY MANAGEMENT OF DIABETES

CHAPTER OBJECTIVE

After studying this chapter, the reader will be able to explain the specific role of nutrition and diet in the overall management of Diabetes Mellitus.

LEARNING OBJECTIVES

After reading this chapter, you will be able to:

1. List the steps in dietary counseling of a patient with diabetes.

2. Identify the primary goals for the patient with various types of diabetes.

3. List the nutritional recommendations by the American Diabetes Association (ADA) for patients with diabetes.

4. Give examples of nutritional interventions necessary for specific situations which occur in diabetes such as illness, hypoglycemia, hyperglycemia, exercise programs, and pregnancy.

INTRODUCTION

Nutrition is one of the cornerstones in the management of diabetes. All individuals with diabetes, regardless of their age, type or severity of diabetes must be made aware of the importance of dietary management. Each patient needs education and counseling by a qualified professional related to diabetes and nutrition. This should include the development of an individualized meal plan based on the goals of management for his/her diabetes and lifestyle.

Food is an important and integral part of everyone's life. Food in this culture is associated with love and rewards. Asking patients to alter their food intake and eating patterns and habits, requires sensitivity and compassion. Simply handing the newly diagnosed person with diabetes a preprinted diet and advising them to go home and "Follow your diet" is to assure failure.

The goal of education and counseling for nutrition is to facilitate the individual's ability to make positive changes in nutritional habits. This involves the use of a "team approach" including the patient, physician, nutritionist, nurse and other health professionals. It is crucially important to involve other family members and significant others in the educational process to foster a family approach to diabetes.

Recent years have brought major revisions to the nutritional management of diabetes. Greater variety in medications, insulin regimes and the advent of self-blood glucose monitoring (SBGM) have allowed increased flexibility in meal plans. Meal plans are higher in carbohydrate and lower in protein than earlier recommendations. There is also a more flexible attitude toward sucrose in the meal plan especially for the patient with type 1 diabetes.

Today's nutritional recommendations for individuals with diabetes are very similar to the recommendations made by national health organizations for all persons to improve overall health through good nutrition. Taken all together, these changes mean that nutrition for persons with diabetes is now more flexible and specific to the individual. With increased ability to comply more fully with their food plan, this will result in the achievement of improved blood glucose control and enhanced health for the person with diabetes.

NUTRITIONAL GOALS

The following are the general goals for individuals with diabetes:

- Establish day to day consistency in eating habits by following an individualized meal plan.

- Consistently achieve as near-normal blood glucose levels as possible.

- Attain optimal blood lipid levels.

- Achieve and then maintain a reasonable body weight.

- Maintain normal growth rate in children and adolescents.

- Provide adequate nutrition to mother and child during gestation and lactation.

- Maintain optimal nutrition to improve overall health.

NUTRITIONAL GUIDELINES

The current nutritional guidelines of the American Diabetes Association are consistent with those of the American Heart Association, National Cancer Institute, U.S. Dietary Guidelines and the National Institute of Health's National Cholesterol Education Program. All rec-

ommendations must be individualized for the specific patient taking into account particular therapeutic needs and goals.

Calories

Energy in the form of calories is necessary for body functioning. Calorie requirements vary through the lifespan and in special circumstances such as pregnancy. After the required amount of calories is determined, adjustments can be made in the food plan to promote weight changes and provide the proper amount of calories for various levels of activity.

Adults

Calorie requirements for adults are established by first determining the height, weight, and activity level of the individual. Calories are prescribed to achieve and maintain desirable body weight (DBW). The DBW is a theoretical weight based on height, sex and body frame size. A quick calculation of DBW can be achieved by allowing 100 lbs for a woman and adding 5 pounds for each inch over five feet. The formula for men is to add 6 pounds for every inch over five feet to 106 pounds. These are for individual with a medium body frame, therefore in both men and women subtract 10% for a small body frame and add 10% for a large body frame. A more exact range is given in *Table 2-1*.

The **maintenance calorie requirements** can be calculated by multiplying the desirable body weight (DBW) in pounds by the following factors:

- Men and physically active women = DBW × 15

- Most women, sedentary men, adults >55yr = DBW × 13

- Sedentary women, sedentary adults >55yrs and obese adults = DBW × 10

Over 80% of all persons with type 2 diabetes are overweight and the major goal of their treatment is to improve glycemic control through caloric reduction leading to weight loss. Weight loss has a definite positive effect on beta cell functioning and insulin sensitivity by increasing the number of receptors on the cellular surface and improving the intracellular metabolism, which are the major problems in the insulin resistance of obesity. The loss of as little as 7 to 10 pounds often improves fasting glucose levels dramatically (Davidson, 1998). With increased physical activity and weight loss the control of the symptoms of diabetes is a strong possibility in most overweight type 2 patients. To promote weight loss, the following are the guidelines:

To lose one pound a week: Multiply DBW in pounds by the calories required for maintenance. Subtract 500 calories from daily requirement and/or increase energy expenditure through exercise. *Ex:* Woman age 37

135 (DBW) × 13 = 1755 cal (Maintenance) - 500 cal = 1,255 cal to lose l/lb/wk

To lose two pounds a week: Follow above but subtract 1,000 calories from daily requirement and/or increase energy expenditure through exercise. For weight gain do the opposite (Nutrition Guide for the Professional, ADA, 1988).

TABLE 2-1
Desirable Weight Ranges—Ages 25 and over*

Height (no shoes) (ft. in.)	Men Weight Range	Men Weight‡ MRW = 100	Women† Weight Range	Women† Weight‡ MRW = 100
4 9			90–118	100
4 10			92–121	103
4 11			95–124	106
5 0			98–127	109
5 1	105–134	117	101–130	112
5 2	108–137	120	104–134	116
5 3	111–141	123	107–138	120
5 4	114–145	126	110–142	124
5 5	117–149	129	114–146	128
5 6	121–154	133	118–150	132
5 7	128–159	138	122–154	136
5 8	129–163	142	126–159	140
5 9	133–167	146	130–164	144
5 10	137–172	150	134–169	148
5 11	141–177	155		
6 0	145–182	159		
6 1	149–187	164		
6 2	153–192	169		
6 3	157–197	174		

*Adapted from the 1959 Metropolitan Desirable Weight table (weight, in pounds, without clothing; height without shoes).

†For women between the ages of 18 and 25, subtract 1 lb for each year under 25.

‡Midpoint of medium frame range used to compute MRW: MRW = [(actual weight)/(midpoint of medium frame range)] × 100.

Source: Krall, L., & Beaser, R. (1989). *Joslin diabetes manual* (p. 52). Philadelphia, Lea & Febiger.

Children

In the first year of life, children require approximately 55 cal/pound of body weight. From one to ten years of age the requirement drops to 36–45 cal/pound. The exact determination is made based on growth charts. It is extremely difficult to maintain any type of constant caloric intake in young children, although most children do consume about the same amount each day. At this age, the main concern is the avoidance of concentrated sweets and assurance of sufficient total caloric intake of a nutritionally adequate diet (Benz and Kohler, 1980).

With the requirement of 15–17 calories per pound, girls in the preteen and teen years require many fewer calories than boys of the same age. Boys from eleven to fifteen years of age require an average of 30 calories per pound and from ages sixteen to twenty the caloric requirement ranges from 15 calories per pound for sedentary boys to 22 calories per pound for very active young men.

Pregnancy

During pregnancy, the caloric needs of the diabetic woman increase as the pregnancy progresses. In the first trimester 13–15 calories per pound are usually needed. During the second and third trimesters the caloric need increases to 16–17 calories per pound. Careful consideration must be given to proper weight gain to ensure adequate fetal growth and to prevent starvation ketosis in the mother. It may be necessary to make adjustments to the calorie level more frequently during pregnancy to assure proper nutrition for both mother and baby. During lactation, the calorie level remains above that needed in the non-pregnant state but should be individually calculated based on weight (Nutritional Guide for Professionals, ADA, 1988). In addition to the total calories consumed, careful attention should also be focused on the daily distribution of calories. The calories should be spread as evenly as possible throughout the meals and snacks. This will help in avoiding a large concentration of calories at any time which could overtax the impaired ability of the person with diabetes to properly metabolize food components and result in poor glucose control. Generally, four to five hours between meals during the day are advised to allow blood sugars to return to premeal levels and also to avoid hypoglycemia due to long intervals between meals.

COMPOSITION OF THE DIET

Carbohydrates

Carbohydrates provide 4 calories per gram. They are the body's major sources of energy. Carbohydrates can be used immediately as a source of energy as blood glucose or can be converted to glycogen and stored in the liver as glycogen through the process of glycogenesis for future glucose needs or converted to triglycerides and stored in the adipose tissues. *SIMPLE CARBOHYDRATES* are called monosaccharides and are found naturally primarily as sucrose, glucose and fructose in fruits and vegetables. These are also the sugars added to foods to enhance sweetness. The crystalline form of sucrose is known as table sugar.

COMPLEX CARBOHYDRATES are also referred to as "polysaccharides" or "starches." They occur naturally in foods such as vegetables, cereals, wheat, rice and corn.

Early diets for diabetes concentrated on severe restriction of carbohydrates. The recommendations today for dietary composition of the diabetic diet, from the ADA, are that carbohydrates compose 45% to 60% of the total calories. It is recommended that the majority of these calories come from the complex carbohydrate group. In the past, patients with diabetes were advised to avoid sucrose because it is rapidly absorbed and raises the blood sugar dramatically. Although this may be true when sucrose is consumed as the sole nutritive component (*ex:* soft drinks, some types of candies) of the food, it is not as much of a problem when taken as part of a mixed meal and spaced throughout the day. Therefore the use of modest amounts of sucrose and other refined sugars may be consumed when taken as part of a mixed meal and spaced throughout the day. This more liberal attitude on sweets has allowed a wider choice of foods and as a side benefit, has increased patient compliance (Davidson, 1998). The foregoing are simply guidelines that must be individualized to the particular patient depending on the impact of the diet on blood glucose and lipid levels as well as considering individual eating habits.

Fiber

Emphasis is placed on ingestion of unrefined and complex carbohydrates which contain fiber. Studies have shown that diets high in natural fiber and carbohydrates, result in a lowering of blood glucose and low-density lipoprotein cholesterol in patients with diabetes (Powers, 1978). The average dietary fiber intake currently found in the adult American diet is 10 to 30 grams per day with an average for men of 19 grams and for women the average is 13 grams. The recommendation of the American Diabetes Association (ADA) is to follow the fiber recommendations for the general public for good health, which is 20–35 grams of fiber per day. Dietary fiber is classified in two types, soluble and insoluble. Both types of fiber promote a feeling of satiety which can aid a weight loss program.

Soluble fiber forms a gel in the gastrointestinal tract and may therefore slow the absorption of glucose and reduce serum lipids. Sources of soluble fiber include legumes, oats, barley, some fruits (such as apples and grapefruit), and vegetables.

Insoluble fibers increase the bulk of the stool and decrease the transient time of the stool. In these ways it is helpful in the prevention and treatment of constipation and has been implicated as beneficial in the prevention of cancer. Good sources of insoluble fiber are whole wheat, wheat, corn bran and some vegetables.

Proteins

Protein is necessary for growth and for body maintenance. It can also be a secondary source of energy. There are several factors which influence the amount of protein that is converted to glucose such as the amount of carbohydrate in the diet, whether the individual is in a fed or fasting state, insulin availability, and the amount of fuel needed for exercise. Protein contributes 4 calories per gram ingested. Food sources of protein include milk, dairy products, meat, soybeans, dried beans, peas, lentils, nuts and seeds.

Protein content in the average diet is commonly 25–35% of total calories consumed. This is probably somewhat more than the amount needed. Early prescriptions for people with diabetes contained recommendations for high levels of protein consumption. Research has since shown that a high protein diet in the individual with diabetes may contribute to deterioration of renal function. A reduction of dietary protein decreases the nitrogen in the urine. Although the ideal percentage of total calories from protein remains in dispute, the current recommendations for persons with diabetes are the same as the Recommended Dietary Allowance (RDA) which is 1 g/kg of body weight for adults. The total protein content of the diet should therefore be about 10–20% of total calories. For most children, adolescents and athletes, 1.2 g/kg will meet the protein needs (Funnell et al., 1998).

Studies have shown that restricting protein in combination with blood glucose and blood pressure control can slow the progression of renal disease. In the presence of overt nephropathy, a protein intake of not less than 0.8 g/kg or 10% of calories is recommended. Levels lower than 0.6 g/kg can lead to protein malnutrition (Funnell et al., 1998).

Fat

Fats are calorie dense, contributing 9 calories per gram. Fats are stored in the body as triglycerides in the adipose tissue. They can also be utilized as an energy source in the form of free fatty acids. Examples of food sources of fat are: meat fats, oils, cheese, salad dressings, gravies, margarine, butter, mayonnaise, whole milk, many of the snack and "quick" or "fast" foods. Methods of cooking such as frying add fats to foods not normally high in fat content. Elevated serum lipid (blood fats) levels, especially high cholesterol levels have been implicated in the development of atherosclerosis (Davidson, 1998).

Arteriosclerotic complications are a major problem for patients with diabetes. Studies have shown that coronary artery disease is reduced in diabetic patients consuming diets high in carbohydrate and low in fat. Because dietary fat can affect serum lipid levels, patients with diabetes are now advised to reduce their fat intake and replace those calories with carbohydrate. The current recommendation by the American Diabetes Association is that fat intake be less than 30% of total calories consumed. Important also is the type of fat consumed and the recommendations are that polyunsaturated fat (vegetable oils such as corn, safflower, soybean, sunflower, cottonseed, and walnuts) should be 10% of total calories, saturated fats (animal fats, coconut and palm oils, high-fat dairy products, hydrogenated vegetable oils) less than 10%, and monounsaturated fats (olive and peanut oil, nuts [except walnuts]) 10–15% of total calories. Dietary cholesterol is found only in animal foods. In some persons dietary cholesterol appears to raise blood cholesterol more than in other individuals. Substituting unsaturated fat sources for saturated fat will help to lower the intake of dietary cholesterol. The recommendation is to reduce dietary cholesterol intake to less than 300 mg/day. Limiting the intake of eggs, cheese, red meats, organ meats and whole milk should decrease cholesterol and saturated fat intake which are the major factors contributing to elevated blood cholesterol levels. Some studies have recently indicated that fish oil supplements may reduce triglycerides and blood cholesterol, but research is still inconclusive and does not allow a definite recommendation (Physician's Guide, ADA, 1988). Because the goal

of less than 30% dietary fat may seem unrealistically low to persons used to very high levels of fat in the diet, any reduction is considered a positive step and the reduction of fat may need to be a phased series of changes in meal planning.

Sodium

The recommended sodium intake for persons with diabetes is less than 3,000 mg/day. This is a modest reduction in intake and is recommended due to the propensity in patients with diabetes for diabetic nephropathy and high blood pressure. For patients with mild to moderate hypertension, sodium intake should be limited to less than 2,400 mg/day (ADA, 1999). Sodium intake can be reduced by limiting the use of table salt, processed and convenience foods.

Vitamins And Minerals

There are no special recommendations for persons with diabetes in regard to vitamins and minerals. Many popular articles have been published recently in regard to the need in diabetes for supplementation of minerals, specifically zinc, chromium and magnesium. Only in the presence of severe deficiency is there an indication that supplementation is beneficial. Studies have shown specifically that supplementation with chromium had no beneficial effect on blood glucose control (Mooradian et al., 1994). There has been no specific recommendation made in regard to these minerals. The response of most diabetes professionals is that it is best to follow a well balanced and nutritionally complete diet until scientific evidence proves that special supplementation is beneficial. For those patients on very low calorie diets to promote weight loss (below 1,000 calories), a physician should be consulted in regard to the need and recommendation for supplementation.

Water

Water does not provide calories, but it is an essential dietary component whose importance is often overlooked. It accounts for one half to three fourths of body weight. Water is important in regulating body temperature, in carrying nutrients to the cells and removing wastes and in all of the body's chemical processes. Drinking 6 to 8 glasses of water per day, in addition to other sources of water in the diet such as beverages and water in food, is the recommended intake.

Other Dietary Considerations

Sweeteners in the Diet

Sweeteners are divided into two categories: nutritive, which contain calories (*ex:* fructose and sorbitol) and non-nutritive, which are counted as noncaloric (*ex:* aspartame, saccharin, Acesulfame-K). The use of both types is acceptable for patients with diabetes. However, moderation in use within established safe levels should be advised. Calories must be included in the food plan. Patients should be encouraged to use a variety of sweeteners to reduce the intake of any one product.

Aspartame - is made from protein and marketed as: Nutrasweet® for use in reduced/calorie and sugar free products and Equal® for tabletop use. It is undesirable for cooking as it will lose its sweetness under prolonged heat.

Saccharin - is a white crystalline powder synthesized from toluene. It is marketed under various names such as "Sweet N'Low"® and "Sweeta"®. Saccharin is heat stable and can be used in cooking. Many people notice a bitter aftertaste with this product. The safety of saccharin has been controversial and the product carries a warning label.

Acesulfame-K - is a derivative of acetoacetic acid and is marketed as "Sweet One"® and "Sunette"®. Food products containing this sweetener are usually reduced in calories. It has no bitter aftertaste and can be used in cooking.

Fructose - is a natural sugar found in fruits and honey. Fructose is marketed for use as "Estee-Fructose"®. One teaspoon contains 16 calories (same as sucrose or "table sugar"). It seems to cause a less dramatic rise in blood sugars after meals and for this reason has been used (Powers, 1978).

Sorbitol - along with fructose is often incorporated into foods such as cake mixes, candy bars and cookies that are technically sugar free but may have as many calories as a non sugar-free product. Sorbitol may also have a laxative effect and cause diarrhea or cramping.

Fat Replacements

Over twenty fat replacements are currently being used in food products (Funnell et al, 1998). They are classified according to the nutrients from which they are made. Carbohydrate sources include modified food starches, cellulose, gums, maltodextrins and dextrins. Protein fat substitutes are from egg whites, milk and texturized proteins. Fat replacements from fat (*ex:* caprenin, salatrim, and olestra) are currently available in foods on the market.

Use of Alcohol

In most cases, it is not necessary for patients with diabetes to abstain from alcohol. However, patients with diabetes should consult their physician before including alcohol in the meal plan. Alcohol is to be avoided if the patient has neuropathy, pancreatitis, unstable diabetes with frequent episodes of hypoglycemia (low blood sugar), or hypertriglyceridemia. If alcohol is permitted, the individual should be provided with specific guidelines regarding alcohol use.

Alcohol should be used in moderation and the recommendation is that persons with diabetes can have up to two drinks of an alcoholic beverage per day (1 drink = 12 oz beer or 5 oz wine or 1½ oz distilled spirits). Alcohol contains 7 calories per gram. In the diet plan, alcohol should be substituted for fat exchanges. One equivalent of alcohol equals two fat exchanges. Sweetened mixers and cordials should be avoided because of their high sugar content.

Alcohol can be absorbed from the stomach or small intestine and is metabolized in the liver. It does not require insulin to be metabolized. It is recommended that alcohol be consumed with a meal or soon after a meal. Hypoglycemia is the major concern for the person with diabetes when alcohol is taken without food. Low blood sugar may occur up to 12–16 hours after alcohol is ingested due to the inhibition of glycogen release from the liver. It is also important to recognize that alcohol raises triglycerides and may potentiate or interfere with the action of other medications.

SPECIAL DIETARY NEEDS

Sick Day Adjustments to Food Plans

Illness, especially when nausea and vomiting occurs, requires that the person with diabetes who is taking insulin or medication to lower blood sugar, make food adjustments. These adjustments and other rules to assure blood glucose control are referred to as sick day management (see Chapter 7). The most important of these guidelines is of course that the individual never discontinue taking their diabetes medication or insulin. Adjustments to dosage may be necessary and medical advice should be obtained.

Consuming fluids is critically important during an illness to prevent dehydration. Soft semi-solid foods and smaller, more frequent meals are generally better tolerated during illness. If regular foods are not tolerated, carbohydrate-containing liquids or soft foods (such as regular soda pop, jello, fruit juices) should be consumed at the calorie level of the meal plan. If fever, vomiting, or diarrhea are occurring, small amounts of salted foods and liquids (broth, vegetables, tomato juice) are important to replace electrolyte loss (see Chapter 7).

Foods from the "Free Food List" can be used after the caloric and carbohydrate content of the individual's meal plan has been met. Developing a sample menu in advance, which is based on the personal meal plan can be very helpful in handling a sick day.

Exercise

For persons with type 1 diabetes, exercise usually requires food and/or insulin adjustments. Since exercise affects each individual differently, the adjustments should be based on checking blood glucose and on the previous experience of the individual with the particular type of exercise. For routine exercise which is done at the same time each day, such as daily walking, the food plan should be adjusted to meet those constant needs. For sporadic exercise, it may be necessary to increase food intake to prevent hypoglycemia during or after exercise. Delayed hypoglycemia presents a problem to some individuals since blood values can continue to decline for up to 12 to 24 hours following exercise (Davidson, 1998).

Persons with type 2 diabetes on diet alone or diet and oral agents will probably not need to make any adjustments. Their goal is often weight loss and the exercise is one of the important factors in promoting this goal.

METHODS FOR TEACHING MEAL PLANNING

A variety of methods are available for teaching the diabetic individual and no single educational tool works in every situation. It is often best to use a variety of methods and tools to allow the patient the optimal chance for understanding and complying with the food plan. Meal planning approaches fall into four categories: (1) basic guidelines, (2) exchange system, (3) counting plans and (4) sample menus.

TABLE 2-2
Carbohydrate and Calorie Content of Foods Appropriate for Sick Day Use

Food Item	Carbohydrate Content (g)	Approximate Calories
STARCH/BREAD EXCHANGES		
1 slice bread	15	80
1/2 cup hot cereal	15	80
6 saltine crackers (2-in squares)	15	80
4 soda crackers (2 1/2-in squares)	15	80
3 graham crackers (2 1/2-in squares)	15	80
1/2 cup ice cream	15	170
(omit 2 fat exchanges)		
1 cup broth soup	15	80
1 cup soup, cream, reconstituted with water	15	125
(omit 1 fat exchange)		
MEAT EXCHANGES		
1/4 cup low-fat cottage cheese	0	65
1 oz. American or Swiss cheese	0	100
1 poached or soft-boiled egg	0	75
VEGETABLE EXCHANGES		
1/2 cup tomato juice	5	25
1/2 cup vegetable juice	5	25
FRUIT EXCHANGES		
1/2 twin popsicle	10	40
Fruit juices: (unsweetened)		
1/3 cup cranberry, grape	15	60
prune juice,	15	60
1/2 cup apple, pineapple,	15	60
apricot,	15	60
1/2 cup cherry, grapefruit,	15	60
orange, peach juice	15	60
MILK EXCHANGES		
1 cup skim milk	12	90
1 cup low-fat milk	12	120
1 cup whole milk	12	150
1 cup yogurt (plain, skim milk)	12	90
1 cup yogurt (plain, low-fat milk)	12	120
1 cup yogurt (plain, whole milk)	12	150
1/4 cup plain pudding	12	70
SIMPLE CARBOHYDRATES		
1/2 cup ice milk	15	125
(omit 1 fat exchange)		
1/2 cup regular gelatin	15	80
1/4 cup sherbet	15	80
4 oz. regular carbonated beverages, cola type	15	55

Source: Reprinted from Kulkarni, K. D. (1987). Altering the basic meal plan. In M. Power (Ed.), *Handbook of diabetes nutritional management* (pp. 187–188), with permission of Aspen Publishers, Inc. © 1987. Data from *Food values of portions commonly used* by J. A. T. Pennington and H. N. Church, J. B. Lippincott, 1980.

Basic Guidelines

The resources used to teach the patient the concepts of basic nutrition, healthy eating and the relationship between diabetes and nutrition are such things as the USDA/HHS (Health and Human Services) Dietary Guidelines, Basic Four Food Groups and Healthy Food Choices.

Exchange System

Exchange Lists for Meal Planning - The exchange system developed by the American Diabetes Association, American Dietetic Association and the Public Health Service is the fundamental tool used in the dietary treatment of diabetes. The exchange list groups similar types of foods into six categories so that when a definite number of each exchange is consumed, a constant number of calories and nutrients is maintained. In addition, a wide variety of food choices is given. The exchange list groups are starch/bread, meat, vegetables, fruit, milk and fat. The foods within each category are interchangeable in the prescribed amounts. For example, in the fruit list one-half cup of orange juice can be exchanged for one- fourth cup of grape juice or half a grapefruit. In the meat group one egg can be exchanged for 1 ounce of cheese or 1 ounce of chicken. The exchange system is easy to learn and provides a highly nutritious, well-balanced diet. An abbreviated

TABLE 2-3

Free Foods

A free food is any food or drink that contains less than 20 calories per serving. You can eat as much as you want of those items that have no serving size specified. You may eat two or three servings per day of those items that have a specific serving size. Be sure to spread them throughout the day.

Drinks:
Bouillon* or broth without
    fat
Bouillon, low-sodium
Carbonated drinks, sugar-
    free
Carbonated water
Club soda
Cocoa powder, unsweet-
    ened (1 Tbsp.)
Coffee/Tea
Drink mixes, sugar-free
Tonic water, sugar-free

Nonstick pan spray

Fruit:
Cranberries, unsweetened
    (1/2 cup)
Rhubarb, unsweetened
    (1/2 cup)

Vegetables:
(raw, 1 cup)
Cabbage
Celery
Chinese cabbage†
Cucumber
Green onion
Hot peppers
Mushrooms
Radishes
Zucchini†

Salad greens:
Endive
Escarole
Lettuce
Romaine
Spinach

Sweet Substitutes:
Candy hard, sugar-free
Gelatin, sugar-free
Gum, sugar-free
Jam/Jelly sugar-free (less
    than 20 cal./2 tsp.)
Pancake syrup, sugar-free
    (1-2 Tbsp.)
Sugar substitutes (saccharin,
    aspartame)
Whipped topping (2 Tbsp.)

Condiments:
Catsup (1 Tbsp.)
Horseradish
Mustard
Pickles* dill, unsweetened
Salad dressing, low-calorie
    (2 Tbsp.)
Taco sauce (3 Tbsp.)
Vinegar

Seasonings can be very helpful in making food taste better. Be careful how much sodium you use. Read the label, and choose those seasonings that do not contain sodium or salt.

Basil (fresh)
Celery seeds
Chili powder
Chives
Cinnamon
Curry
Dill

Flavoring extracts
    (vanilla, almond, walnut,
    peppermint, butter,
    lemon, etc.)
Garlic
Garlic powder
Herbs
Hot pepper sauce
Lemon

Lemon juice
Lemon pepper
Lime
Lime juice
Mint
Onion powder
Oregano
Paprika
Pepper

Pimento
Spices
Soy sauce*
Soy sauce* low-sodium
    ("lite")
Wine, used in cooking
    (1/4 cup)
Worcestershire sauce

*†3 grams or more of fiber per exchange   *400 mg or more of sodium per exchange*

Source: Reprinted with permission from *Exchange lists for meal planning* (p. 22) (1988). Copyright © by the American Diabetes Association, Inc.

version of the exchange list appears in this text. A complete list of foods and explanation for using the exchange system is found in *Exchange Lists for Meal Planning* by the American Diabetes Association and American Dietetic Association. A list of "free" foods which may be consumed and are not counted in the food plan is included *(Table 2-3).*

Counting Plans

Calorie Counting - This approach is most useful with patients whose goal is weight loss. A baseline calorie level is established and a list of

foods with caloric values is used to make the food plan.

Total Available Glucose (TAG) - A food plan is made based on the anticipated conversion of the food groups to glucose. This allows greater flexibility of food planning and is often used by individuals on intensive insulin management regimes.

Point System - This system uses simplified guidelines for counting the per meal, per snack and total daily intake of calories. For example, one point equals 75 calories (a slice of bread is 1

TABLE 2-4

Suggested General Guidelines for Making Food Adjustments for Exercise for Persons with IDDM*

Type of Exercise and Examples	If Blood Glucose is	Increase Food Intake by	
One hour of moderate activity: *Examples:* swimming, jogging, tennis, gardening	100 to 180 mg/dl	15 g CHO	1 fruit or 1 starch exchange
	180 to 300 mg/dl†	Not necessary to increase food	
	Over 300 mg/dl†	Don't exercise until control is better	
Strenuous activity of 1–2 hour duration *Example:* athletic events	100 to 180 mg/dl	25 to 50 g CHO	1/2 sandwich with milk, or fruit
	180 to 300 mg/dl†	15 g CHO	1 fruit or 1 starch exchange
	Over 300 mg/dl†	Don't exercise until control is better	

*SBGM is essential for all persons in order to determine their exact carbohydrate needs. Persons with NIDDM usually do not need an exercise snack. During periods of exercise, individuals need to increase fluid intake.

†Some individuals will experience hyperglycemia with pre-exercise values around 250 mg/dl.

Source: Reprinted from Franz, M. J. (1987). Exercise and Diabetes Mellitus. In M. Power (Ed.), *Handbook of diabetes nutritional management* (p. 82) with permission of Aspen Publishers, Inc. © 1987. Adapted from *Diabetes and exercise: Guidelines for safe and enjoyable activity* by M. J. Franz, p. 6, with permission of International Diabetes Center, © 1985.

point) and a 1,200 calorie diet equals 16 points. It can also be used for counting other nutrients (e.g., fat, sodium, fiber, carbohydrate, protein).

Carbohydrate Counting - This system is frequently utilized by those on the insulin pump to balance insulin with the amount of carbohydrate eaten. One unit of insulin is usually taken for every 12–15 grams of carbohydrate contained in the meal. In the exchange lists starches/breads contain 15 grams carbohydrate (CHO), vegetables have 5 grams CHO, fruits have 15 grams CHO, milk 12 grams CHO, fats and meats have 0 grams CHO.

Sample Menu Plans

Utilizing sample menus is a simplified approach to meal planning. It is most often used for the patient who has difficulty making food choices and does not require variety in meals.

Individualized Sample Menus - This involves a cycle of menus being prepared in advance to be rotated by the patient. This approach can be used for the client who finds learning a system such as the exchange list too complicated or cumbersome.

Preplanned Menus - Five separate booklets entitled Month of Meals have been developed by the ADA. Each booklet contains 28 days of complete menus and recipes for breakfast, lunch, dinner and snacks. Menus are for 1,500 kcal daily with instructions for adjusting the caloric level up or down.

Food Label Reading

The 1995 food labeling regulations by the FDA and Department of Agriculture expanded mandatory nutrition labeling to almost all food products and provide a standard format for food labels. This label information is very helpful in the various meal planning methods. For instance in carbohydrate counting, the number of grams of carbohydrate is stated right on the label. Calorie content per serving, fat content, and fiber content are areas of helpful information for all individuals concerned with meal planning.

NUTRITIONAL COUNSELING

Before nutritional counseling can begin, certain information must be gathered. DBW and caloric needs must be calculated. It is important to assess current food intake, dietary habits and customs. This can most easily be done through a twenty-four hour dietary recall and interviewing the patient about food preferences.

There are two distinct phases in nutritional education and counseling. The first step which is the initial education occurs at the time of diagnosis or when a change in diabetes management such as switching form oral medications to insulin occurs. The skills learned at this time may be only focused on "survival skills" necessary for the individual to function until more in-depth education can occur. These include basic meal planning and nutrition principles, managing unplanned exercise and the recognition and treatment of hypoglycemia. The second phase is the in-depth or continuing education which is at a more comprehensive level. This would include information required to make decisions to reach management goals, foster self-care, and problem-solving skills that allow a more flexible lifestyle. The skills learned in this phase include such special issues as meal planning for exercise, illness, use of alcohol, restaurant eating, and adjustments for late or delayed meals.

DEVELOPING A NUTRITIONAL CARE PLAN

The nutritional care plan should always be a joint endeavor by the patient/family and the nutrition counselor. The following steps are recommended for an effective plan.

Gather referral information prior to consultation:

- Laboratory data (A1c, Lipid levels, Glucose levels, Renal function)
- Blood pressure
- Medical history and current medications
- Patient limitations on exercise or activity

Assess the patient for the following:

- Height, weight, desired weight
- Clinical signs and symptoms
- Food/nutrition history
- Learning style, cultural heritage, religious practices, food related beliefs, attitudes and concerns and socioeconomic status

Design a nutritional care plan:

- Utilize tools and system of meal planning best suited to patient/family
- Instruct use of food/exercise and blood glucose diary

Evaluate and adjust nutritional care plan:

The plan is always in a state of evolution and should be adjusted as often as necessary to aid the patient in achieving optimal health goals.

TABLE 2-5
Diabetic Exchange Lists

MILK *(12 g carbohydrate, 8 g protein, 0 fat, 80 kcal)*

1 cup nonfat milk	1 cup 2% milk (omit 1 fat exchange)
1 cup yogurt	1 cup whole milk (omit 2 fat exchanges)
1 cup buttermilk	

VEGETABLES *(5 g carbohydrate, 2 g protein, 0 fat, 25 kcal)*

1/4 cup asparagus	1/2 cup eggplant	1/2 cup rhubarb
1/2 cup cabbage	1/2 cup green pepper	1/2 cup string beans
1/2 cup carrots	1/2 cup mushrooms	1/2 cup tomatoes
1/2 cup celery	1/2 cup onions	1/2 cup turnips

FRUIT *(15 g carbohydrate, 0 fat, 40 kcal)*

1 apple	1/2 banana	1/2 cup grapefruit juice
1 tangerine	1/2 grapefruit	1/2 cup pineapple
1 orange	1/2 mango	1/2 cup applesauce
1 fig	2 T raisins	1/2 cup orange juice
1 nectarine	1/2 cup berries	

BREAD *(15 g carbohydrate, 2 g protein, 0 fat, 70 kcal)*

1 slice white bread	1 biscuit
1 slice whole-wheat bread	5 crackers
1 slice pumpernickel bread	8 french-fried potatoes
1 slice raisin bread	1/3 cup corn
1/2 hamburger bun	1/3 cup lima beans
1/2 English muffin	1/2 cup green peas
1 tortilla	1/2 cup potatoes

MEAT *1 oz (7 g protein, 3 g fat, 55 kcal)*

Low fat	1 oz beef, lamb, pork, veal, poultry, fish;
	1/4 cup cottage cheese
Medium fat	Omit 1/2 fat exchange
High fat	Omit 1 fat exchange
	1 oz Cheddar cheese
	1 frankfurter

FAT EXCHANGE *(5 g fat, 45 kcal)*

1 tsp margarine, oil, butter, mayonnaise	6 walnuts
1 T heavy cream, cream cheese	20 peanuts
1 strip bacon	5 olives

Source: Guthrie, H. (1986). *Introductory nutrition.* St. Louis: Mosby.

EXAM QUESTIONS

CHAPTER 2
Questions 10–18

10. Which of the following dietary fibers is most likely to slow absorption of ingested glucose?

    a. Whole wheat

    b. Legumes

    c. Wheat bran

    d. Corn bran

11. In terms of exchanges, $\frac{1}{2}$ cup of peas is equal to which of the following?

    a. One vegetable exchange

    b. One starch/bread exchange

    c. One vegetable and one fat exchange

    d. A free food

12. An example of a noncaloric sweetener is

    a. Dextrose.

    b. Tryptophan.

    c. Aspartame.

    d. Fructose.

13. How many calories are provided by 15 grams of a carbohydrate?

    a. 15

    b. 135

    c. 60

    d. 110

14. What is the recommended caloric distribution of carbohydrates (CHO), protein, and fat in the meal plan for a patient with diabetes?

    a. CHO 45–60%, protein 10–20%, fat up to 30%

    b. CHO 40–45%, protein 30–35%, fat up to 30%

    c. CHO 35–40%, protein 35–40%, fat 35–40%

    d. CHO 25–35%, protein 45–50%, fat up to 25%

15. Which of the following oils is a source of polyunsaturated fats?

    a. Palm

    b. Olive

    c. Peanut

    d. Safflower

16. Patients with diabetes who drink a moderate amount of alcohol should be given instructions on how to avoid which of the following complications?

    a. Ketoacidosis

    b. Hyperglycemia

    c. Hypoglycemia

    d. Cirrhosis

17. What is a basic principle in deciding on an approach for meal planning?

   a. All approaches are based on the exchange system.

   b. The approach should be structured.

   c. Learning the caloric value of foods is essential.

   d. A variety of educational tools may be used to convey understanding.

18. To lose one pound a week, how many calories must be subtracted daily from caloric needs?

   a. 200 calories

   b. 1,000 calories

   c. 500 calories

   d. 100 calories

CHAPTER 3

EXERCISE AND DIABETES

CHAPTER OBJECTIVE

After completing this chapter, the reader will be able to explain the benefits of and guidelines for exercise for patients with diabetes.

LEARNING OBJECTIVES

After studying this chapter, the reader will be able to:

1. Identify four benefits of exercise for patients with diabetes.

2. Specify the normal physiologic response to exercise and how it is altered in patients with diabetes.

3. Indicate the four components of an exercise prescription.

4. Recognize three risks of exercise for patients with diabetes.

5. Specify appropriate measures to avoid or minimize risks of exercise in patients with diabetes.

6. Indicate the effect of exercise on blood glucose levels in patients with diabetes.

INTRODUCTION

Exercise has been considered one of the three main techniques for treating diabetes since the discovery of insulin in 1921. In fact, E. P. Joslin (1959) listed exercise as one of the three main components of diabetes treatment in the Joslin emblem. Before then, exercise as a treatment had been controversial. In an effort to control the signs and symptoms of diabetes, children with the disorder often were forbidden by their physicians to exercise. For these patients, being treated as "sickly" increased their feelings of isolation and depression. Fortunately, today's health professionals recognize the valuable contribution of exercise to people with diabetes. Several well-known sports figures, including the tennis player Bill Talbert, the triathlete Bill Gilbert, and the baseball players Catfish Hunter and Ron Santos, have shown that people with diabetes can succeed in all forms of exercise-related activities.

The specific benefits, risks, precautions, and appropriate prescription guidelines for exercise have only recently been defined for patients with diabetes. Today, exercise is viewed as an integral and focal point of achieving optimal control of blood glucose levels, decreasing the risks of complications, and promoting a feeling of well-being.

PHYSIOLOGIC RESPONSE TO EXERCISE

In intense exercise, the demand by the muscles for glucose increases greatly. Despite an up to 20 times increase in the demand in glucose uptake by the exercising muscles, the body is able to maintain normal levels of blood glucose. Understanding how the body compensates in diabetes requires knowledge of the mechanisms of homeostasis in people without diabetes.

Response in People Without Diabetes

To meet the increased energy requirements of exercise, both cardiovascular and metabolic responses are needed to ensure delivery of oxygen and fuel to the exercising muscles. The combination of increases in respiration and cardiac output, redistribution of blood flow, and an increase in capillary perfusion to the muscles results in increases in oxygen supply to the tissues and in the removal of carbon dioxide. Fuel to maintain normal levels of blood glucose comes from the utilization of glucose at the cellular level and from an increase in the production of glucose in the liver through glycogenolysis and gluconeogenesis. The increased production of glucose is due to a decrease in insulin secretion and an increase in the secretion of catecholamines, growth hormones, glucagon, and glucocorticoids.

In the resting state, muscle obtains only 10% of its energy requirements from glucose. Almost 90% of the energy comes from the oxidation of fatty acids. During exercise, the following changes occur:

- At the onset of exercise (first 5–10 minutes), the primary use of fat as fuel changes to the use of glycogen stored in muscle. The rapid breakdown of these stores causes a buildup of the by-product lactic acid. With continuing exercise, blood flow increases. Levels of lactate decrease as glucose is taken up from the circulation and aerobic metabolism is established.

- Uptake of glucose from the muscles increases to 7–20 times greater than uptake in the resting state in the next 10–40 minutes of exercise. During the first 40 minutes, about three fourths of the glucose is derived from glycogenolysis (breakdown of liver glycogen to glucose) and about one fourth from gluconeogenesis (conversion of lactate, glycerol, and amino acids to glucose).

- As the glucose stored in the liver is depleted, gluconeogenesis increases and accounts for as much as 50% of glucose production in the later stages of exercise.

- Use of free fatty acids or fat for energy during exercise increases with the duration of exercise. Exercise of low-to-moderate intensity results in greater use of fat for fuel. In exercise sessions lasting longer than 2 hours, fat provides the majority of energy. However the oxidation of lipids can never fully replace the use of glucose by the exercising muscle, and muscular fatigue or exhaustion occurs when glycogen stores are depleted.

- After exercise, insulin stimulates the uptake of glucose by the exercised muscles to replenish the depleted glycogen stores. The glycogen stores in the liver are also replaced. This replenishment may take 24–48 hours (Ellenberg & Rifkin, 1983).

Aerobic and Anaerobic Exercise

Theoretically, as long as the demand for metabolic fuel does not exceed the supply, exercise could continue indefinitely. When the intensity increases and the fuel supply can no longer meet the demand, exercise (now anaerobic) can continue for only a short time. The point at which supply exceeds demand is the separation between aerobic and anaerobic exercise. This anaerobic threshold usually occurs between 70% and 85% of maximal heart rate in healthy people. To remain below the anaerobic threshold, a person must exercise at "conversational intensities." At this level of exercise intensity, a person can carry on a conversation without excessive shortness of breath (Davidson, J., 1986).

Response in People with Diabetes

The physiologic response to exercise in patients with diabetes whose blood glucose levels are well controlled and who do not have ketone production is similar to the response in people without diabetes. These patients use blood glucose, glycogen, and free fatty acids during exercise and because of better body utilization of insulin, may be able to reduce the amount of insulin they require. However, if diabetes is not well controlled, changes in metabolism occur that are not seen in people without diabetes. The hormonal and metabolic responses to exercise depend on the degree of blood glucose control at the beginning of exercise.

If a person has a high blood glucose level and ketone production due to lack of insulin before he or she begins to exercise, the result of exercise may include a further increase in plasma glucose, free fatty acids, and ketone bodies (Davidson, J., 1986). The mechanism by which this increase occurs is as follows: (1) Lack of insulin prohibits entry of glucose into cells. (2) Stimulation of secretion of counterregulatory hormones in response to cellular lack of glucose results in increased levels of glucose and free fatty acids. (3) High levels of free fatty acids lead to an increase in the production of ketone bodies.

Sufficient insulin is necessary for the proper metabolic response to exercise in both diabetic and nondiabetic people. It is crucial to recognize that exercise cannot substitute for insulin and that exercising when blood glucose levels are high and ketones are present can be dangerous.

A more common problem for patients with diabetes who are taking insulin is hypoglycemia due to exercise. Insulin inhibits the production of glucose from the liver. When a person without diabetes begins to exercise, hepatic production of glucose increases because of a decrease in insulin secretion. Because injected insulin continues to be absorbed during exercise, the level of insulin in the circulation increases. This higher level inhibits the hepatic production of glucose that would normally be used to supply glucose for the muscles. The result is a decrease in blood glucose levels to less than normal, and the exerciser experiences hypoglycemia. Hypoglycemia can also be delayed (up to 24 hours) after exercise sessions. This delay is due to an increased sensitivity of muscle tissue to insulin as a result of exercise and the increase in glucose uptake by muscles and liver to replenish glycogen stores depleted during the exercise. Hypoglycemia occurs much less often in patients who use oral hypoglycemic agents or who control diabetes by diet and exercise (Davidson, J., 1986).

EXERCISE IN TYPE 1 DIABETES

For several reasons, exercise is beneficial to patients with type 1 diabetes. However, guidelines must be followed and precautions taken to maximize the benefits, minimize the risks, and ensure safety.

Benefits

The benefits of exercise include the following:

- An improvement in glucose tolerance occurs because of the increase in glucose utilization and insulin sensitivity. A smaller amount of insulin is required to stimulate the uptake of glucose in exercising muscle than is needed in resting muscle. The more prolonged effect of exercise on glucose is the decrease in the fluctuation of blood glucose levels over the next 24 hours due to the uptake of glucose to replenish stores of glycogen. The improvement in overall blood glucose levels is indicated by an improvement in the levels of glycosylated hemoglobin (Lebowitz, 1991).

- A reduction in insulin dosage is facilitated, because exercise potentiates the lowering of blood glucose levels.

- The risk of coronary heart disease is reduced. Regular aerobic exercise can reduce the serum level of low-density lipoproteins and increase the level of high-density lipoproteins. The risk of coronary heart disease is greatly increased in patients with diabetes. Autopsy studies in patients 19–38 years old with type 1 diabetes showed that in patients in whom the onset of diabetes occurred before the age of 15, significant coronary disease had already occurred at the time of death (Stein, Goldberg, Kalman, & Chesler, 1984). The well-known Framingham Study on cardiac risk factors confirmed that diabetes is an independent risk factor for coronary atherosclerotic disease.

- Weight control is facilitated. Attaining and maintaining desirable body weight may help in maintaining normal levels of blood glucose by promoting insulin sensitivity. Body fat is decreased, and lean body mass is preserved.

- Both diastolic and systolic blood pressures are decreased. High blood pressure potentiates all the long-term problems associated with diabetes.

- The exerciser's sense of well-being and self-image are improved. A feeling of accomplishment accompanies the completion of an exercise session.

Precautions and Risks

Patients should take certain precautions when exercising and should be aware of the risks associated with exercise.

- For anyone with type 1 diabetes, the first step in starting an exercise program should be a complete history and physical. This is particularly true if the person is more than 30 years old or has had diabetes longer than 10 years.

- An exercise stress electrocardiogram is recommended for all patients over the age of 35. The results will help detect those who may have silent ischemic heart disease or an exaggerated hypertensive response to exercise or who are at risk for postexercise orthostatic hypotension.

- Exercise can cause worsening of long-term complications of diabetes. Patients should be screened for these before they begin an exercise program and should choose appropriate activities *(Table 3-1)*. For example, exercise may result in retinal or vitreous hemorrhage in patients with proliferative retinopathy. Exercises that increase the blood pressure (heavy lifting or those associated with Valsalva-type maneuvers) are especially dangerous and should be avoided by these patients. Jarring or rapid head movement during exercise could cause hemorrhage or retinal detachment.

- Exercise also increases the risk of soft-tissue and joint injuries in patients with peripheral neuropathy. Peripheral sensitivity and circulation should be evaluated. Patients with peripheral neuropathy or decreased circulation should avoid exercises that could cause foot trauma. Patients with autonomic neuropathy may be vulnerable to dehydration or postural hypotension. Also, the ability to engage in high-intensity exercise is impaired because of the decrease in maximum heart rate and aerobic capacity. In patients with diabetic nephropathy, exercise is also associated with an increase in proteinuria. It is not known whether the proteinuria has any long-term effect on kidney function, but it may cause patients to be concerned.

- Vigorous exercise is also contraindicated in patients with poor metabolic control of diabetes. When blood glucose levels are significantly elevated (greater than 300 mg/dl), strenuous exercise may increase the level further and initiate or increase production of ketones, resulting in serious consequences. Exercise programs should be postponed until hyperglycemia is adequately controlled.

TABLE 3-1

Exercise Precautions for Diabetic Patients with Medical Complications

Complication	Precaution
Insensitive feet or peripheral vascular insufficiency	Avoid running. Choose walking, cycling, swimming.
Active proliferative retinopathy	Avoid exercises associated with increased intraabdominal pressure, Valsalva-like maneuvers, or acceleration-deceleration trauma to the head.
Hypertension	Avoid heavy lifting and Valsalva-like maneuvers. Choose exercises that involve the lower- rather than primarily upper-extremity muscle groups.

Source: Sperling, M. (Ed.). (1988). *The physician's guide to insulin-dependent (type I) diabetes: Diagnosis and treatment* (p. 56). Copyright © 1988 by the American Diabetes Association, Inc.

- Exercise can increase the risk of hypoglycemia. Exercising when insulin is at its peak of action or for extended periods without adequate carbohydrate replacement can result in a severe hypoglycemic event. Additionally, delayed hypoglycemia may occur for as long as 12–18 hours after the workout ceases. Also, certain drugs, such as ß-blockers, aspirin, and alcohol, can increase the risks of hypoglycemia.

Guidelines for Safe Exercise

Table 3-2 summarizes guidelines for safe exercise for patients with type 1 diabetes. Other considerations include the following:

- The primary consideration is adequate metabolic control. When blood glucose control is poor or has fluctuated greatly, several serious risks are associated with strenuous exercise. The accepted guideline is to avoid exercise when the blood glucose level is 300 mg/dl or more, especially when ketonuria is present. In this situation of insulin deficiency, the production of glucose and the breakdown of fat to ketones exceed the ability of the muscles to use the ketones. The result is ketosis and ketoacidosis. If the blood glucose level is less than 100 mg/dl, a food supplement before exercise is recommended to avoid hypoglycemia during the exercise session (see chapter 2).

- Blood glucose monitoring is an essential component of exercise. Monitoring glucose levels before, during, and after an exercise session can help the patient ascertain how exercise affects these levels. Keeping records of the blood glucose level and the time, type, and intensity of exercise is important so patterns can be used to adjust food and insulin intake.

- The timing of exercise has several implications. It would be simple to adjust diabetes management for exercise if the exercise occurred at the same time with the same intensity and duration each day. On a practical level, this scenario is not only unrealistic but also undesirable. Various changes in blood glucose levels occur normally during the day. For example, exercise later in the day might cause a greater drop in blood glucose level than exercise before or after breakfast. Ideal timing for preplanned exercise is 1–3 hours after breakfast, when postprandial levels of blood glucose tend to be at the highest. Peak times for insulin action should be avoided.

- The exercising limbs of the body should not be used as sites for the injection of insulin. The abdomen is the preferred site before total body exercise. When an exercising limb is used for insulin injection, the increase in circulation to that area could cause more rapid and complete

---

TABLE 3-2
Guidelines for Safe Exercise for Patients with Type I Diabetes

All patients should do the following when exercising:

• Carry an identification card and wear a bracelet at all times that indicates they have diabetes.

• Be alert for signs of hypoglycemia during and for several hours after exercise.

• Have immediate access to a source of readily absorbable carbohydrate (such as glucose tablets) to treat hypoglycemia.

• Drink sufficient fluids before, after, and, if necessary, during exercise to prevent dehydration.

• Measure blood glucose levels. Take appropriate action if the level is less than 80 or more than 240 mg/dl by color estimation or more than 300 mg/dl with a meter.

Source: Sperling, M. (Ed.). (1988). *The physician's guide to insulin-dependent (type I) diabetes: Diagnosis and treatment* (p. 56). Copyright © 1988 by the American Diabetes Association, Inc.

---

absorption of insulin and an increased risk of hypoglycemia.

• Exercise may require adjustments in the meal plan. It is important to recognize that patients may overcompensate in supplementing the diet before exercise and that this overcompensation could result in reducing the benefit of exercise to overall glucose control. The most effective way to determine how much extra food is needed is to monitor blood glucose levels before, during, and after exercise. If the exercise is of low intensity and short duration and the blood glucose level is more than 100 mg/dl, there is usually no need for additional food. For more vigorous exercise of longer duration, the preexercise snack should be based on the blood glucose level and the time of action of previ-ously injected insulin. For this type of exercise, an additional 15–30 grams of carbohydrate snack should be eaten for every 30–60 minutes of exercise (see chapter 2).

• Consumption of an adequate amount of fluids before, during, and after exercise is crucial to safe exercise. Patients who have diabetes often are preoccupied with the importance of replacing carbohydrates and forget that water is the most important nutrient lost during exercise. Water is essential to provide a source for cooling perspiration and to avoid dehydration.

• An adjustment in the insulin dosage may be needed when strenuous exercise (e.g., marathon run, triathlon event) of long duration is planned. The usual methods involve decreasing the insulin that will be acting during the activity by 10–20% (Franz, 1985). For these more involved adjustments, consulting with a physician is strongly recommended.

• Extremes in environmental temperature can increase the drop in blood glucose during exercise. In extreme heat or cold, the body must increase the rate of energy expended to maintain temperature homeostasis. To avoid hypoglycemia, patients should wear loose-fitting clothing when exercising in hot temperatures and layer clothing for cold temperatures. Exercising in a temperature-controlled environment during weather extremes is recommended.

• Use of proper equipment for exercise is important to ensure safety. Equipment such as exercycles and treadmills should be in good condition and appropriate for the person exercising. Clothing and footwear are also important. Good athletic shoes are important to reduce foot injuries, which are a special concern in patients with diabetes. Before exercise, the feet should be carefully examined for areas of redness or pressure.

- During exercise, patients with diabetes should carry identification and a source of fast-acting carbohydrate (e.g., glucose tablets, Lifesaver® candies, raisins). Whenever possible, patients with diabetes should exercise with someone who knows that they have diabetes and is familiar with the appropriate measures to follow in a diabetic emergency.

EXERCISE IN TYPE 2 DIABETES

The characteristics of type 2 diabetes are decreased insulin binding at the receptor sites, increased insulin resistance, and hyperinsulinemia. The typical patient with this kind of diabetes is a good candidate for an exercise program. Obesity and inactivity are often contributory factors for the development of diabetes in this patient. If the proper guidelines are followed, the benefits can far outweigh the potential risks.

Benefits

The benefits of exercise in patients with type 2 diabetes include the following:

- Exercise is an important part of a weight control program. With exercise and a reduction in the number of calories consumed, a healthy weight loss can be attained. It is usually not necessary for patients on this type of program to supplement exercise with food to prevent hypoglycemia.

- In many cases, regular exercise in addition to a weight loss program can control type 2 diabetes. Because working muscles use insulin more effectively, blood glucose control is improved. Exercise leads to enhanced sensitivity to insulin. Consequently, the metabolism of carbohydrates and lipids is improved, and the result is improved glucose tolerance.

- Exercise enhances the body's sensitivity to insulin, and plasma levels of insulin are decreased. Hyperinsulinemia has been suspected as a risk factor in the development of atherosclerosis and coronary artery disease. The lower levels of insulin in the bloodstream reduce this potential risk and may help prevent macrovascular complications.

- Dosages of insulin or oral hypoglycemic medication can often be reduced and in some cases eliminated through a program of regular exercise and weight control.

- Exercise may also reduce the risk of coronary heart disease by improving the serum lipid and lipoprotein profiles. Exercise reduces the serum levels of low-density and very low-density lipoproteins, cholesterol, and triglycerides and increases the levels of high-density lipoprotein, which is thought to protect against cardiovascular disease. In addition, regular exercise lowers the blood pressure and cardiac work both during the exercise and at rest. This effect is extremely important in patients with type 2 diabetes because of the multitude of risk factors usually present in this population.

- Additional benefits include an enhanced quality of life and an improvement in the sense of well-being. Many patients report a reduction in stress and a feeling of accomplishment when they exercise regularly, which contributes to a feeling of good health.

Precautions and Risks

The precautions and risks listed for patients with type 1 diabetes also apply to patients with type 2 diabetes. However, because those with type 2 are still producing insulin, their blood glucose levels are not as unstable during exercise as those of patients with type 1, who produce little or no insulin. Other precautions and risks include the following:

- Prolonged or vigorous exercise can potentiate the hypoglycemic effects of oral hypoglycemic agents and insulin. In these instances, supplementary food may be needed to prevent hypoglycemia. The timing of food intake can be changed to coincide with exercise periods to prevent an increase in the total number of calories consumed and to promote the weight-loss benefits of exercise.

- Patients with type 2 diabetes are usually older, are often overweight or frankly obese, and may have significant long-term complications. For these patients, starting a safe exercise program may be difficult.

- Patients with type 2 diabetes should be carefully assessed for atherosclerotic heart disease. Exercise could precipitate arrhythmias and myocardial ischemia or infarction. These patients should have a stress electrocardiogram before they begin an exercise program. Referral of patients with known cardiac problems to a cardiac rehabilitation exercise program that can provide close supervision and necessary monitoring is an excellent way to ensure maximal safety.

- In obese patients, injuries to the ligaments occur more often and degenerative joint disease may be worsened by some types of exercise.

Guidelines for Safe Exercise

The guidelines for safe exercise for patients with type 2 diabetes are similar to those for patients with type 1 diabetes.

- Exercise should not be attempted when blood glucose levels are out of control. In type 2 diabetes, the problem is not ketoacidosis, but rather a profound dehydration and disturbance in electrolyte balance that can occur with continued elevation in the level of blood glucose. Monitoring of blood glucose levels and keeping records are indispensable components to ensure the success and safety of an exercise program.

- Many patients who have type 2 diabetes have been sedentary for several years. Because they are deconditioned and cannot exercise continuously for any length of time, a program of gradually increasing exercise is most successful and safest.

EXERCISE FOR WEIGHT REDUCTION

Exercise is often used as an adjunct to diet in promotion of weight loss. Increased physical activity increases energy expenditure (*Table 3-3*) and may help in weight reduction. When a person is sedentary, energy expenditure for physical activity accounts for approximately 30% of calories. In an exercise program, this amount can be increased to 45–50%. Physical exercise alone usually does not result in significant loss of weight, but it may increase muscle mass and decrease body fat. Calorie restriction combined with exercise is an excellent method of promoting weight loss. In patients with diabetes, it is important to ensure that the weight reduction diet contains sufficient carbohydrate to maintain muscle glycogen stores.

Exercise In Diabetes and Pregnancy

In the past, women with diabetes often were counseled to avoid exercising during pregnancy. The primary reason was the fear that exercise could harm the fetus. Today, women who exercised regularly before their pregnancy can usually continue their exercise program during the pregnancy.

With the correct timing of exercise to balance food and insulin action, exercise can be an important aspect of diabetes management to facilitate optimal blood glucose control. Target heart rates for exercise during pregnancy have not been established. A heart rate at approximately 50% of the woman's target rate when she is not pregnant is usually advised and is thought to be adequate to improve glucose utilization.

TABLE 3-3
Energy Expenditure for Household, Recreational, and Sport Activities

ACTIVITY	TIME NEEDED TO USE 250 CALORIES	CALORIES USED PER HOUR OF ACTIVITY
Rest and light activity		
(50–200 calories per hour)		
Lying down or sleeping	3 hrs. 8 min	80
Sitting	2 hrs. 30 min	100
Driving an automobile	2 hrs	120
Fishing	1 hr. 50 min	130
Standing	1 hr. 45 min	140
Domestic work	1 hr. 23 min	180
Moderate activity		
(200–350 calories per hour)		
Bicycling (5 1/2 mph)	1 hr. 10 min	210
Walking (2 1/2 mph)*	1 hr. 10 min	210
Gardening	1 hr. 8 min	220
Canoeing (2 1/2 mph)	1 hr. 4 min	230
Golf	1 hr	250
Lawn mowing (power mower)	1 hr	250
Bowling	55 min	270
Lawn mowing (hand mower)	55 min	270
Rowboating (2 1/2 mph)	50 min	300
Swimming (1/4 mph)	50 min	300
Walking (3 1/4 mph)	50 min	300
Dancing (slow step)	50 min	300
Softball	45 min	325
Badminton	40 min	350
Horseback riding (trotting)	40 min	350
Square dancing	40 min	350
Volleyball	40 min	350
Rollerskating	40 min	350
Vigorous Activity		
(over 350 calories per hour)		
Mini-trampoline	38 min	400
Ditch digging (hand shovel)	38 min	400
Shoveling	38 min	400
Ice skating (10 mph)	38 min	400
Wood chopping or sawing	38 min	400
Tennis, singles	35 min	420
Waterskiing	32 min	460
Dancing (fast step)	30 min	490
Jogging	26 min	585
Skiing (downhill)	25 min	600
Squash and handball	25 min	600
Soccer	25 min	600
Singles racquetball	20 min	775
Skiing (cross-country)	15 min	900
Running (10 mph)	15 min	900

*Walking or jogging = 100 calories per mile: cover 2.5 miles to use 250 calories.
Source: Learning to live well with diabetes (p. 61). (1987). DCI Publishing.

In women with gestational diabetes, mild aerobic exercise does not seem to have an adverse effect on either mother or fetus. For many women with gestational diabetes, a low-intensity exercise program three to four times a week could be suffi-cient to improve glucose control and reduce the need for insulin.

The Exercise Prescription

The key to a successful exercise program is the patient who must carry it out. A specific prescription for exercise should be designed with the full participation of the person for whom it is intended. The steps in designing an individualized exercise prescription are as follows:

1. Obtain medical clearance from the patient's physician that lists any restrictions or precautions to be taken.

2. Determine with the patient the goals for the program, including weight loss, improvement of blood glucose control, etc.

3. Establish the amount of time the patient can commit to the program.

4. Interview the patient about preferred exercise activities.

5. Plan with the patient the specifics of the exercise program.

The components of an exercise prescription are type, intensity, duration, and frequency of exercise. The specific goals in each of these areas should be determined on the basis of the patient's age, lifestyle, stage of physical conditioning, and motivation.

Type

The goal of an exercise program is to achieve optimal cardiovascular, muscular, and metabolic response to aerobic exercise. The word aerobic literally means "with oxygen." In aerobic exercise, the need for large amounts of oxygen to convert glucose or glycogen to pyruvic acid and adenosine triphosphate (ATP) for muscle work is met by an increase in cardiac output with only a small increase in blood pressure. Aerobic exercise is characterized by prolonged submaximal exertion, and activities should be low resistance and high movement.

Recommended modes of aerobic exercise include walking, swimming, cycling, jogging, and dancing. These involve contractions of large muscle groups in a continuous or rhythmical manner. If there are no contraindications, the type of exercise can be a matter of personal preference. Exercises that may place the patient at risk for foot injury, such as jogging and running, should be limited in patients with peripheral neuropathy. Body-contact sports or those that involve heavy lifting or a head-down position should be avoided by patients with proliferative retinopathy.

Anaerobic exercise is characterized by maximal or near-maximal exercise of short duration. The ability of the heart and lungs to provide oxygen to muscles increases the amount of lactic acid, which is accumulated, and exhaustion sets in quickly. Weight lifting and sprinting are examples of anaerobic activities that also produce a significant increase in blood pressure.

Intensity

It is important for patients to know how intense the exercise should be. If the intensity is too low, the exercise may be of little benefit. If the intensity is too high, the activity may not provide any additional health-related benefits, and in patients with vascular disease, the resultant increase in blood pressure and cardiac output could be harmful.

A graded exercise test may be helpful in determining a patient's exercise tolerance. The pulse rate based on the results of this test may provide the most information for intensity of exercise. In order to obtain the maximum cardiovascular and pulmonary benefits from an exercise program, the heart must reach and maintain the target heart rate. A target rate can be determined from the maximal heart rate obtained through the graded exercise test. The zone is between 50% and 75% of the maximal heart rate. However, patients with diabetes are often unable to attain these goals and may have as much as 15–20% lower achievable maximal heart rates.

Pulse rates should be taken for 10 seconds and multiplied by 6 periodically throughout the exercise. On the basis of this information, the patient can then adjust the intensity of the exercise. The lower end of the zone is the recommended goal at the start of a program. The target heart rate should be increased progressively over a period of weeks, with the exercise increasing in intensity as tolerated by the patient.

Another method of determining target heart rate is to subtract the patient's age from 220 and multiply that number by the percent intensity recommended for the patient. This number divided by 10 would then be the 10-second or target heart rate *(Table 3-4)*.

Peripheral neuropathy in the fingers or use of ß-adrenergic blocking agents may make the pulse rate an inaccurate measure of exercise intensity. A more practical method of assessing the intensity is the patient's ability to speak during the exercise. If the patient cannot talk while exercising, the intensity is too high; if he or she can sing, the intensity is too low.

Duration

Duration is the length of time the exercise is done at the target heart rate without stopping. The duration time does not include warm-up and cool-down time, only the aerobic part of the exercise session. A duration of not less than 20–30 minutes at the target heart rate intensity is necessary to ensure beneficial effects of the exercise.

At the start of an exercise program, short periods of rest of 1–2 minutes during the session are encouraged. The patient can gradually increase to continuous exercise without breaks. For patients whose goal is weight reduction, extending the exercise duration to more than 40 minutes will

TABLE 3-4

Target Heart Rates During Exercise: Heart Beats per 10 Seconds

Intensity *Age*	15	20	25	30	35	40	45	50	55	60	65	70
60%	20	20	19	19	18	18	17	17	16	16	15	15
75%	25	25	24	23	23	22	22	21	20	20	19	19
85%	29	28	27	27	26	25	25	24	23	22	22	21

Source: Franz, M. J. (1985). *Diabetes and exercise: Guidelines for safe and enjoyable activity* (p. 13). International Diabetes Center.

increase the utilization of fat stores expended during exercise.

Patients who have been sedentary should begin with a duration at which they can maintain the prescribed intensity of exercise. The rule of thumb would be to add 1–5 minutes of duration per week, depending on the patient's ability to progress.

Frequency

Frequency refers to the number of times a week that the exercise is performed. In order to achieve the cardiovascular and pulmonary benefits of exercise, a minimum of three to four times a week is needed. Weight control benefits are most often achieved by exercising five to six times a week. Because the beneficial effects of exercise rapidly disappear after only a few days without exercising, the recommendation is to allow no more than 2 days of rest between sessions.

The Exercise Session

Each exercise session should begin with a 5- to 10-minute warm-up session of flexibility or stretching exercises to help prepare the body for more vigorous activity and to reduce the risk of musculoskeletal injury. This part should begin with an initial circulatory warm-up, because muscles should not be stretched when cold.

The higher intensity part of the exercise session at the target heart rate is then done according to the exercise prescription. Patients who start from a low level of fitness should check their heart rate 5-10 minutes after starting the exercise to ensure that they are remaining within the guidelines.

A cool-down period of 10–12 minutes should follow to end the session and allow the body to return gradually to a resting state. A recovery heart rate of less than 100 beats per minute should be achieved before the session ends.

EXAM QUESTIONS

CHAPTER 3
Questions 19–27

19. For patients with type 2 diabetes, which of the following steps is best to help ensure beneficial effects from exercise?

    a. Increase insulin dosage.

    b. Increase caloric intake.

    c. Monitor urinary levels of ketones frequently.

    d. A physical exam or stress test

20. With adequate circulating insulin, which occurs after exercise to replenish glucose stores?

    a. A decrease in insulin sensitivity.

    b. An increase in glucose uptake by the exercised muscle.

    c. An increase in insulin secretion.

    d. A decrease in the mobilization of free fatty acids from adipocytes.

21. For patients with type 2 diabetes, exercise training appears to enhance which of the following?

    a. Sensitivity to insulin

    b. Turnover of beta cells

    c. Pancreatic secretion of insulin

    d. Catecholamine response

22. What are the four basic components of an exercise prescription?

    a. Intensity, duration, target heart rate, and frequency

    b. Quality, quantity, mode, and aerobic activity

    c. Intensity, quality, mode, and duration

    d. Intensity, duration, frequency, and type

23. Which of the following is the most appropriate exercise for a person with severe peripheral neuropathy in the lower extremities?

    a. Jogging

    b. Running

    c. Swimming

    d. Football

24. Which of the following is a method of preventing exercise-induced hypoglycemia?

    a. Testing the urine for ketones

    b. Eating food supplements after the exercise

    c. Avoiding exercise when insulin levels are lowest

    d. Adjusting the dosage of insulin

25. When the blood glucose level is greater than 300 mg/dl and ketones are present in the urine, exercise will probably do which of the following?

    a. Decrease blood glucose and ketone levels

    b. Increase blood glucose and ketone levels

    c. Have no effect on blood glucose and ketone levels

    d. Improve insulin action

26. What is the end product of fat metabolism?

    a. Epinephrine

    b. Carbohydrate

    c. Lactic acid

    d. Ketone bodies

27. On the basis of the information in Table 3-4, what is the suggested target heart rate in beats per minute for a 40-year-old patient who is exercising at 75% intensity?

    a. 132

    b. 122

    c. 112

    d. 92

CHAPTER 4

PHARMACOLOGIC THERAPIES
IN DIABETES

CHAPTER OBJECTIVE

After completing this chapter, the reader will be able to discuss the current medications used as therapy for diabetes, listing mechanism of action and indications and guidelines for useage.

LEARNING OBJECTIVES

After studying this chapter, the reader will be able to:

1. Recognize the mechanism of action of oral antidiabetes agents.

2. Differentiate between the actions of oral antidiabetes medication.

3. Recognize the action times of various types of insulin.

4. Indicate guidelines for proper insulin administration, mixing, and storage.

5. Specify the most common complication of insulin therapy.

6. Indicate the proper use of and correct administration technique for glucagon.

INTRODUCTION

Medications are the third major component in the management of diabetes. For those with type 1 diabetes, insulin is an absolute necessity. Without insulin replacement, they cannot survive. The discovery of insulin in 1921 by two young Canadian physicians was a landmark, not only in diabetes but in all of medicine. It truly was a life-saving discovery.

For patients with type 2 diabetes, the development of a treatment that can be taken by mouth was an exciting advance. Before the availability of pills for diabetes in 1951, patients with known or suspected type 2 diabetes avoided seeking medical care that could result in their being prescribed insulin. Many sought better management of their diabetes when they knew that oral medications were available.

The use of insulin and oral antidiabetic medications is known as combination therapy and has allowed for better glucose control in selected patients.

The availability of glucagon is another life-saving development in diabetes care. Patients feel more confident when they have a readily available resource in case of a hypoglycemic emergency.

Many patients with diabetes have concurrent health problems. It is important to understand the interactions and possible contraindications for other medications that the patient is taking.

ORAL ANTIDIABETES AGENTS

What are oral antidiabetes agents? An important fact for patients to know is that the agents are not insulin. Insulin is a protein that can be taken parenterally only. It would be destroyed by gastric secretions if taken orally. Oral antidiabetes agents are effective only in those patients with diabetes who continue to secrete insulin.

Patients with type 2 diabetes have insulin resistance in addition to impairments of insulin action and hepatic glucose production. Treatment is targeted at these problems and to decreasing the rate of digestion of carbohydrates. Five groups of medications are now available to treat these alterations in glucose control.

It is important to emphasize again and again that the most important therapy for patients with type 2 diabetes is appropriate diet and exercise. Unfortunately, this method may be overlooked and unnecessary amounts of medication used instead. With sulfonylureas and meglitinides too much medication exacerbates hyperinsulinemia and probably hyperlipidemia, which may contribute to vascular illnesses (Chisholm, 1994).

Sulfonylureas

When research was being done on the use of sulfonamides in the 1940s, it was noted that the most frequent side effect in laboratory rats was hypoglycemia. Subsequently, a group of drugs with the specific action of reducing hyperglycemia, known as sulfonylureas, was developed and used clinically in the mid 1950s. This group of antidiabetic agents, which are known as oral hypoglycemic agents due to their action in directly lowering the blood sugar, is the most widely prescribed for use in type 2 diabetes today.

Mechanism of Action

One of the primary modes of action of sulfonylureas is on the beta cells of the pancreas. Therefore, for these drugs to work, the pancreas must still be capable of producing insulin. The direct pancreatic effect of stimulating insulin secretion is thought to be the most prevalent mode of action in the first few weeks to months of therapy (Davidson, J., 1998). Secondary effects include improved action and numbers of insulin receptors on muscle and fat cells, improved glucose transport at the postinsulin receptor sites and a reduction in glucose production from the liver (Funnell et al., 1998).

First-Generation Sulfonylureas

The first-generation sulfonylureas are given in larger doses than the second generation of these drugs.

Tolbutamide (Orinase®). Tolbutamide is a short-acting sulfonylurea that is usually taken two to three times a day. It is metabolized in the liver and excreted in the urine. It is the least potent of the drugs in this group, and for this reason, it is often considered safer than the others for the elderly and patients with renal impairment. Recommended Dose: 0.25–3.0 grams in divided doses.

Acetohexamide (Dymelor®). Acetohexamide is an intermediate-duration drug that is usually taken one to two times a day. It is metabolized in the liver to an active metabolite that has more than twice the potency of the original compound. Some patients who cannot use tolbutamide can control their diabetes with this medication. The drug is excreted through the kidney. Recommended Dose: 0.25–1.5 grams in single or divided doses.

Tolazamide (Tolinase®). Tolazamide is an intermediate-duration sulfonylurea. It is taken once or twice a day and has diuretic activity. It is metabolized by the liver to be less active than its parent compound and is excreted by the kidney. Few side effects occur with this drug. Recommended Dose: 0.1–1.0 grams single or divided doses.

Chlorpropamide (Diabinese®). Chlorpropamide is the most potent of the first-generation hypoglycemic agents. It has an extremely long half-life of up to 72 hours and is taken only once a day. It is metabolized partially in the liver, and a significant part is excreted unchanged. It must be used with caution in the elderly and in those with kidney disease. It can cause water retention and hyponatremia by potentiating the effect of antidiuretic hormone. The length of action of chlorpropamide has been the cause of severe and prolonged hypoglycemia in the elderly. Also patients who take this drug may experience the "Antabuse" (disulfiram) effect (facial flushing) when they drink alcohol. Recommended Dose: 0.1–0.5 grams in single dose.

Second-Generation Sulfonylureas

The second-generation sulfonylureas were approved for use by the U.S. Food and Drug Administration in the 1980s. These compounds are 100 to 200 times more potent than the first-generation drugs, and the doses are much smaller (e.g., milligrams). Because a wide range of doses can be used, it is not necessary to switch medications if a patient requires a small adjustment in dosage. The second-generation agents have fewer side effects and are less likely to interact with other medications.

Glyburide (DiaBeta®, Micronase®, Glynase PresTab®). Glyburide is metabolized in the liver to inactive metabolites and excreted 1:1 in urine and bile. This pattern of excretion may make it useful in patients with renal disease. The duration of action is 24 hours, and the drug is given in single or divided doses. Glyburide has a sustained effect on blood glucose levels during the night because of its duration of action; the result is a pronounced lowering of the fasting blood glucose level. It also has a more pronounced effect than glipizide in lowering hepatic production of glucose. This difference may result in more nocturnal hypoglycemia with this drug than with glipizide. It should be used with caution in the elderly. Recommended Dose: 1.25–20 mg in single or divided doses.

Glynase PresTabs are available in 3- and 1.5-mg tablets. This formulation of glyburide increases the bioavailability (percentage of drug that is actually available for use) of the drug for improved absorption, and it can be divided easily to allow greater ease in drug titration (Upjohn, 1992). Recommended Dose: 0.75–12 mg in single or divided doses.

Glipizide (Glucotrol®, Glucotrol XL®). Glipizide is metabolized in the liver to nonactive metabolites and is excreted primarily in the urine, with some excretion in the bile. This drug should be taken on an empty stomach. The duration of action is 12–18 hours. It should be used with caution in the elderly. Recommended Dose: 2.5–40 mg single or divided doses. Single dose for XL.

Glimepride (Amaryl®) is the newest sulfonylurea. It is taken once daily with the first meal of the day. Amaryl is used alone and in combination with insulin. Recommended Dose: 1–4 mg in single dose.

Side Effects

Sulfonylureas are well tolerated, and the prevalence of side effects is low. Gastrointestinal disturbances occur in approximately 5% of all cases. These include a feeling of fullness, heartburn, anorexia, nausea with occasional vomiting, and flatulence. Rashes such as erythema and pruritus, which are usually transient, occur in about 2% of patients. Other side effects include hematologic reactions, antithyroid activity, and diffuse pulmonary reactions. Unwanted weight gain is also a common side effect.

Chlorpropamide is associated with the most side effects. It causes the disulfiram effect (facial flushing, headache) in 35% of patients. Chlorpropamide also occasionally causes water retention and hyponatremia because of an enhancement of the effects of antidiuretic hormone.

Hypoglycemia is the major complication associated with use of sulfonylureas. It is more pronounced with the use of Diabinese (chlorpropamide) and, to a lesser extent, Glucotrol because of their longer duration of action. Other risk factors for hypoglycemia are alcohol intake, poor nutrition, gastrointestinal disease, impairment of renal function, and drug interactions. The elderly are most susceptible to hypoglycemia because of tendencies to eat erratically or skip meals.

Biguanides

A group of drugs known as biguanides (phenformin, buformin, and metformin) were in widespread use as antidiabetic agents until the 1970s. Because of an association between these medications and the development of fatal lactic acidosis, biguanides were banned in the United States in 1977.

The U.S. Food and Drug Administration again approved the use of metformin (Glucophage®) as safe for treatment of type 2 diabetes in 1994. The mechanism of action of this drug is less clear than that of the sulfonylureas (Bailey, 1992). Some slowing of carbohydrate absorption occurs, and conversion of glucose to lactate in the gastrointestinal tract increases. In addition, the rate of glucose production in the liver is reduced. Insulin secretion is not increased, and decreases in levels of low-density lipoprotein and increases in the levels of high-density lipoprotein have been reported. Metformin does not promote weight gain in obese patients; in fact, it has shown to promote weight loss.

Metformin is usually taken before meals in divided doses of 500–3,000 g/day. It is excreted unchanged via the kidneys.

Side Effects

The most common side effects of metformin are gastrointestinal, including loss of appetite, nausea, and diarrhea. These may occur when a patient first starts taking the drug and usually disappear after the first few doses. Lactic acidosis is extremely rare, but it can occur, especially in patients with impaired liver or renal function. Metformin should not be used in these patients. It rarely causes hypoglycemia when used alone.

Alpha-Glucosidase Inhibitors

At present only one medication, Acarbose (Precose®) is available in this group. It delays carbohydrate absorption in the gastrointestinal tract. In high dosages, this drug can cause malabsorption syndrome. Precose reduces the increase in the concentration of blood glucose that occurs after meals by delaying or preventing absorption of the ingested carbohydrate. The initial dosage is 25 mg before meals. The maximum dose is 100 mg before each meal.

Side Effects

The most pronounced side effects of precose are bloating, flatulence, and diarrhea. Starting with a low dose and working up to a higher dose usually minimizes side effects. Hypoglycemia may also occur, especially when this drug is used in combination with a sulfonylurea.

Thiazolidinediones

These medications work primarily to reverse insulin resistance. Because they do not increase insulin secretion, they do not cause hypoglycemia. It is recommended that they be taken with meals. They can be used alone as monotherapy, but are most often used in combination with sulfonylureas or insulin. When used with insulin a lower dose of insulin is usually required. Rosiglitazone

(Avandia®) and Prioglitazone (ACTOS®) are the two medications approved for use. Troglitazone (Rezulin®) has been taken off the market due to reported cases of liver damage.

Side Effects

Hepatic dysfunction is a concern with this medication and therefore patients must be very closely monitored with liver function testing. Patients should report symptoms of liver damage including nausea, vomiting, abdominal pain, fatigue, anorexia or dark urine. Hypoglycemia occurs only when this medication is used in combination therapy.

Meglitinides

Repaglinide (Prandin®) has a similar action to the sulfonylureas in increasing the release of insulin from the pancreas and is considered, because of this, to be a hypoglycemic agent. This drug has a rapid onset, a very short duration of action and a minimal potential for accumulation. These attributes minimize the incidence of hypoglycemia. Recommended Dose: 0.5–16 mg in divided doses right before main meals.

Side Effects

Hypoglycemia can occur with this medication, particularly when meals are skipped. Patients should be cautioned not to take the dose if the meal is skipped. Other reported side effects include headache and gastrointestinal disturbances.

Selection of Patients

Patients most suited to the use of oral antidiabetic agents are those who are obese, are more than 40 years old, and have stable type 2 diabetes of less than 5 years' duration. Patients who previously used insulin should have required less than 40 units/day to achieve stable control. Use of oral antidiabetic agents is not recommended as a substitute for dietary and exercise management, and these two methods should be tried before drugs are used (Funnell et al., 1998).

Contraindications

Oral antidiabetic agents are not suitable for patients with the following conditions:

- **Type 1 diabetes** or a tendency to ketoacidosis.

- **Allergy to sulfonylurea compounds.**

- **Pregnancy or lactation.** The effect of oral antidiabetic agents on the fetus and newborn is unknown. Women who are attempting to become pregnant or who are unsure of when they might become pregnant should also avoid these compounds. Therefore, use of these agents by women in their child-bearing years is usually contraindicated.

- **Major surgery, serious infection, trauma, acute myocardial infarction.** These are situations of high stress in which oral antidiabetic agents are often ineffective in controlling high blood glucose levels.

- **Impaired hepatic or renal function.** These drugs are metabolized in the liver, and most are excreted by the kidney. Serious episodes of hypoglycemia or worsening of renal function can occur in patients with poor kidney or liver function.

Sulfonylureas and Cardiovascular Changes

In the early 1970's, the University Group Diabetes Program reported the results of a study done with the drug tolbutamide. The report indicated that patients who took this drug had higher risk of dying of heart disease than patients who did not. Many physicians question the results of the study for several reasons, including the large number of people with preexisting heart disease who were selected to take the drug.

After much controversy, most medical organizations did not accept the findings, and the oral agents remain in use. Package inserts for all oral antidiabetic agents now include information on this study and on other potential problems. The inserts state that diet and exercise are the first modes of treatment and that medications should be used only if these modes have "clearly failed."

Drug Interactions

Several drugs potentiate the hypoglycemic action of the sulfonylureas. These include alcohol (impairs hepatic gluconeogenesis), ß-adrenergic blockers (e.g., propranolol), large doses of salicylates (greater than 2 g/day), and sulfonamides. Other drugs such as thiazide and loop diuretics, estrogens, and glucocorticoids antagonize the therapeutic effects of sulfonylureas and increase blood glucose levels.

Starting Use of Oral Antidiabetic Agents

After the most appropriate agent is selected for the patient, the lowest effective dose is prescribed. Gradual increases are made to obtain the desired control. Chlorpropamide is used only with caution in the elderly. The second-generation agents are usually the agents of choice today. They interact less often with other medications and have fewer side effects and alternative routes of excretion. Using a single daily dose when possible is thought to increase patients' compliance with treatment.

Drug Failure

About two-thirds of the patients who start using oral antidiabetic agents achieve good control of their blood glucose levels. If the oral agents are not effective within a 1-month trial, the result is considered a primary failure, and insulin needs to be considered. In some patients, oral antidiabetic agents may be effective for a time and then lose effectiveness. This situation is called secondary failure, and generally insulin is required to control blood glucose levels.

In both cases, physicians may try a second medication before making the switch to insulin therapy. "Human failure" may play a large part in both sets of patients if they erroneously assume that diabetes can be controlled by medication alone without the proper efforts in diet and exercise.

COMBINATION THERAPY

The use of oral antidiabetic agents and insulin together is called combination therapy. The combination of a medication which addresses one of the other metabolic problems with insulin often results in better glucose control. The use of oral antidiabetic agents with insulin may result in the need for only one injection (rather than multiple injections) of insulin a day. The advantages of this kind of therapy include the simplicity of the regimen and possibly increased safety from hypoglycemia with greatly improved glycemic control (Bingham & Riddle, 1989).

INSULIN

Until the 1980's, insulin was extracted from the pancreases of cows and pigs. In its early form, it contained a number of impurities. It was necessary to inject a large amount of fluid to deliver small doses of insulin. Only regular insulin was available, and because it lasted only 6–8 hours, three or four injections per day were necessary. The needles were large and also rapidly became dull, making injections painful. Syringes made of glass had to be boiled to maintain sterility. The injections caused ugly skin changes, and the impurities in the insulin often caused allergies and insulin resistance. When resistance occurred, the dose had to be increased to larger amounts.

Today highly purified insulins, which cause fewer skin reactions and changes, are available. Human insulin, developed in the 1980's, has decreased the prevalence of insulin resistance. Disposable syringes and needles of much smaller size have made the injection of insulin almost painless.

Insulin Secretion

Insulin is a hormone secreted by the beta cells of the pancreas. It is a protein and therefore must be injected for use. The body's normal physiologic secretion of insulin is of two types: (1) continuous or basal secretion of insulin to take care of the needs throughout the day; and (2) bolus secretion in response to ingestion of food. The best control of diabetes occurs when those two actions of insulin are most closely imitated.

Insulin preparations have four major characteristics:

1. **Source.** Initially, only insulin derived from beef or pork or a combination of these two sources was available. Animal insulins differ in protein structure from human insulin. Beef insulin differs at three amino acid sites. Pork insulin is structurally more similar to human insulin; it differs at only one amino acid site. Because of this difference, beef insulin causes more antigenic responses than pork insulin does, and the beef-pork combination is thought to be the most antigenic.

    Human insulin and the human insulin analog (lispro) is manufactured through the use of recombinant DNA technology (biosynthetic) and is identical in structure to the insulin made by the human pancreas. It has many advantages and only a few disadvantages *(Table 4-1)*. Because human insulin is less immunogenic (antibody inducing) than animal insulins, it is recommended for patients who only require short-term use of insulin during periods of illness or stress. Human insulin is recommended for all patients whose diabetes is newly diagnosed, who are taking insulin for the first time, who are pregnant, or who are having difficulty with animal insulins (Campbell, 1988; *Table 4-2)*. Human insulin is absorbed slightly faster and acts more quickly than animal insulins. Because of the better absorption, patients may

---

TABLE 4-1
Advantages and Disadvantages of Human Insulin

Advantages

*   Human insulin is the least immunogenic insulin preparation available.

*   Human insulin causes the formation of fewer insulin antibodies.

*   Human insulin is absorbed slightly faster and acts more quickly than animal insulins.

*   Biosynthetic and semisynthetic human insulin are safe, effective, and chemically identical to human insulin produced by people without diabetes.

*   Biosynthetic human insulin ensures an unlimited supply of insulin.

*   Human insulin causes less production of IgG antibodies.

*   Human insulin is usually less expensive than purified pork insulin.

*   Some physicians think that biosynthetic human NPH insulin may have a different shorter pattern of action from other NPH insulins. Careful research studies, however, have yet to prove this.

*   Human Ultralente provides a pattern of action of insulin not previously available.

*   Human insulin is not contraindicated in any type of patient with diabetes.

Disadvantages

*   Human insulin is more expensive than conventional insulin.

*   Human insulin is susceptible to frosting.

Source: Campbell, K. (1988, July/August). *Practical pharmacology: Human insulin.* Practical Diabetology, p. 23.

TABLE 4-2
Patients Who Should Use Human Insulin

- Patients with insulin resistance (using more than 100–200 units/day)

- Patients with insulin allergy (local cutaneous reactions, rashes, etc.)

- Patients with lipoatrophy or lipohypertrophy

- All patients with type 2 diabetes and patients without diabetes who are using insulin for a short period or intermittently (e.g., during surgery, infections, total parenteral nutrition)

- All women with type 1 diabetes who are pregnant

- All women with gestational diabetes who use insulin

- All patients with newly diagnosed type 1 diabetes and patients who are taking insulin for the first time

- Possibly, patients receiving intensified insulin therapy

- Vegetarians, Moslems, Hindus, Orthodox Jews, and others who refuse to use beef or pork insulins

Source: Campbell, K. (1988, July/August). Practical pharmacology: Human insulin. *Practical Diabetology,* p. 22.

---

be able to slightly lower the dose. There are no contraindications for human insulin.

2. **Type.** Insulins are classified as rapid acting, short-acting, intermediate-acting, or long-acting; there are also combinations of these. These classifications refer to insulin action times *(Table 4-3),* which includes the onset (how long before the insulin begins to work), the peak (the maximum effect of the insulin), and the duration (how long the insulin will work in the bloodstream).

Rapid acting or lispro acts very rapidly and is clear in appearance. Its onset of action is 15 minutes or less and it peaks in about an hour. This helps to prevent high post prandial glucoses. Its duration of action is only 3–4 hours. Lispro should be injected immediately before a meal and meals should not be delayed. Because it leaves the blood stream so quickly, there is less chance of delayed hypoglycemia. Lispro is available only by prescription.

Regular, or crystalline, insulin is short-acting and is a clear fluid. The onset of action is 30 minutes to 1 hour. The peak occurs in 2–4 hours, and the duration of therapeutic action (dependent on source) is only 6–8 hours. Regular insulin is used alone (especially in intensive insulin management, in illness as sliding-scale insulin, and with insulin pumps) or in combination with one of the intermediate- or long-acting insulins.

NPH and Lente are intermediate-acting insulins. They are cloudy in appearance and have nearly identical action times. The onset of action of human intermediate-acting insulins is 2–4 hours (animal intermediate-acting, 4–6 hours). The peak occurs in 6–8 hours (animal 8–14 hours), and the duration of action can range from 10 to 24 hours.

The only long-acting insulin currently in use is Ultralente. Its onset of action is 4–6 hours. Because this insulin essentially has no substantial peak, it is often used as a background or basal insulin. The duration of action for Ultralente is 18–36 hours. It is cloudy in appearance. Manufacture of PZI, another long-acting insulin, was discontinued in 1991 because of a decrease in usage.

Two combinations of insulin are also available. Novolin 70/30 is a combination of 70% intermediate- and 30% short-acting insulins (e.g., 10 units of 70/30 insulin = 7 units of NPH and 3 units of regular insulin). Also recently made

TABLE 4-3
Onset Peak and Duration of Human Insulins

Insulin	Onset (h)	Peak (h)	Therapeutic Duration (h)	Phamaceutic Duration (h)
Rapid Acting (Lispro Insulin)	<15–30 min	1–2	3–4	
Short Acting (Regular Insulin)	$^1/_2$–1	2–4	6–8	5–12
Intermediate Acting (NPH or Lente)	2–4	6–8	10–16	16–24
Long Acting (Ultralente)	6–8	Minimal	24–36	36+

available is 50/50 insulin, which is a combination of 50% intermediate- and 50% short-acting insulins.

3. **Purity.** Purity of insulin is based on the amount of noninsulin pancreatic proteins in the preparation. The amount of proinsulin present is used to reflect purity, and insulins are defined as purified if they contain less than 10 ppm (parts per million) of proinsulin. Ten years ago, many of the available insulins had 2,000 ppm of proinsulin. Today, all the insulins sold in the United States and most of the Western countries are highly purified and meet the purity standards (Lebowitz, 1991).

The order of purity, from most pure to least pure, is human, pork, beef, and beef-pork combinations. The improvement in insulin purity has had several therapeutic effects. Allergic reactions, lipodystrophy, and lipoatrophy are much less of a problem than before, and stable control can usually be achieved with smaller doses of insulin.

4. **Concentration.** The concentration of insulin refers to the number of units in 1 ml of fluid. U-100 insulin has 100 units/ml and 1,000 units in a 10-ml vial. At one time, insulin came in four strengths: U-40, U-80, U-100, and U-500. U-80 was discontinued several years ago. U-40

was discontinued in the United States in late 1991, but it is still used in other countries. The simplification of products is a definite advantage in minimizing possible confusion in dosing, dispensing and administration of insulin.

U-500, a very concentrated insulin, is not often used. It is used primarily by patients with a high degree of insulin resistance. Because of its potency, U-500 is available only by prescription. The implantable insulin pump uses U-400 insulin, which is not available for purchase by consumers.

If a person is traveling and needs insulin, U-40 may be the only insulin available. Patients should be taught how to draw up the correct dosages in their syringes.

Insulin Administration

Administration of insulin requires use of the correct insulin preparation and equipment, proper storage of insulin, and the consistent use of correct and proper technique.

Storage

It was previously recommended that insulin could be stored at room temperature (less than 80°F [27°C]), away from direct heat and light, if the entire contents are used within 1 month. More sensitive assays have shown that insulin stored at room temperature for 1 month can lose about 1.5% of its potency (Holcomb, 1995). Therefore, whenever possible, insulin should be stored under refrigerated conditions. If the temperature is more than 100°F (37°C), the stability of the insulin begins to deteriorate rapidly. Insulin should never be left in an automobile trunk or glove compartment, where temperatures are often high. If there is any question about the temperature, the insulin should be refrigerated. All unopened vials should also be refrigerated but not frozen. Cold insulin should be brought to room temperature before it is injected, because injection of cold insulin tends to be more painful, and absorption rates can be affected.

Cartridge vials (those used with penlike syringe devices), or prefilled pens either unused or used (punctured), may be stored at room temperature for the following amounts of time: regular or lispro insulin for 28 days; 70/30 insulin mixture for 7 days; and NPH for 14 days (Funnell et al., 1998). As stated earlier, ideal storage is under refrigeration.

Availability of Insulin

Availability of insulin and equipment varies, so patients should carry all insulin and needed supplies with them when they travel. Because of the variances in both temperature and availability, the medication and supplies also should not be kept in a car or checked through with baggage.

Spare bottles of insulin and extra syringes should be kept on hand in case of breakage or loss. Insulin is available without a prescription; however, syringes and needles may require a prescription from a physician. This depends on the state of residence, no perscription is needed for syringes or needles in Texas.

Tips on Insulin Use

Tips on insulin use include the following:

* Patients should always inspect the label of the insulin container to make sure that they have the correct type of insulin and that the expiration date is current.

* They should check the vial of insulin carefully for sediment or other changes visible before withdrawing the insulin into the syringe. Any cloudiness or discoloration of clear insulin; clumping or flocculation (frosting); or failure of NPH, Lente, or Ultralente insulins to remain uniformly suspended is an indication that the insulin should be returned to the pharmacy and not used.

* Consistency in taking insulin at the same time each day is important in achieving better control of blood glucose levels. Meal times should also be consistent, and for patients taking intermediate- or long-acting insulin, the interval between meals should be no longer than 4–5 hours.

Mixing Insulin

When regular insulin is mixed with a suspended preparation of insulin, the regular insulin should always be drawn into the syringe first ("clear before cloudy"). This method avoids the possibility of contaminating the short-acting regular insulin with longer acting insulin and altering the regular insulin's action time.

Lente, and Ultralente insulins can be mixed in any ratio, and the mixtures are stable for 18 months. Prefilling of syringes is acceptable.

Regular insulin plus NPH is the most common mixture of short- and intermediate-acting insulins. The effect of these two insulins combined in one syringe is the same as that of regular and NPH insulin injected separately (Anderson & Campbell, 1990). Prefilled and refrigerated syringes are stable for at least one month.

If regular and Lente insulins are mixed, they should either be mixed and used immediately, or they should be mixed and allowed to interact for 24 hours before they are used. The resultant mixture does not have as rapid an action as the immediately mixed injection. Therefore, when prefilled syringes are being used, it is important not to introduce freshly filled syringes into the treatment regimen. Care givers who make up a 7- to 14-day supply of syringes should always include an extra day's worth of syringes. This practice ensures that the patient will not have to use a freshly prepared syringe whose insulin activity would differ from the activity of the other syringes.

If the prefilled syringes contain an insulin suspension (e.g., NPH, Lente), the syringe must be adequately rotated or rolled to resuspend the insulin before use. In order to prevent insulin crystals from settling down and clogging the needle, prefilled syringes should never be stored vertically, with the needle down.

Site of Injection

Several factors may affect the absorption of insulin and consequently the effects of the insulin on blood glucose levels. The site of most rapid absorption is the abdomen. Next, in order, are the arm, the leg, and the hip. Intramuscular injections of insulin are absorbed faster, and the duration of action is shorter. Exercise of the injected muscle immediately before or after the injection also results in faster absorption and a shorter duration of action. Massaging the injection site or applying heat to the area increases the rate of blood flow through the tissues and causes much more rapid absorption and action from a dose of insulin.

The sites of injection should be rotated within an area (e.g., the abdomen). An injection site should not be used more often than once every 15 days. Repeated injections in the same spot may lead to unsightly lumps or tissue changes, which can cause variable absorption of insulin and fluctuations in blood glucose levels.

Insulin should be injected deep into the subcutaneous layer. Patients should avoid using a 1-in. (2.54 cm) area around the navel and any areas of

large blood vessels or scarring. The angle of the injection depends on the amount of subcutaneous tissue. Generally, pinching up a roll of tissue and injecting at a 90° angle achieves this goal.

Injection Equipment

U-100 disposable insulin syringes are available with attached needles in three sizes: The 1-ml syringe holds 100 units of insulin and has marks indicating 2-unit increments. The $^1/_2$-ml syringe (commonly called Lo-Dose) holds 50 units, and the $^3/_{10}$-ml syringe holds 30 units. Both of the smaller syringes are marked in 1-unit increments, which increases accuracy for measuring odd-numbered doses, and the numbers are larger and more easily read than those on the 1-ml syringe. The syringes come with attached needles in lengths of $^1/_2''$ and $^5/_{16}''$ and needle gauges of 28–30. A special coating on the needle is designed to make insertion easier and less painful.

Reuse of Syringes

Because of the cost of diabetes management, many patients reuse syringes. The position of the ADA is that syringes can be safely reused with the following precautions:

Manufacturers of disposable syringes recommend that they be used only once, because the sterility of a reused syringe cannot be guaranteed. However, some individuals prefer to reuse a syringe until its needle becomes dull. Most insulin preparations have a bacteriostatic additive that inhibits growth of bacteria commonly found on the skin. For many patients, it appears both safe and practical for the syringe to be reused. The syringe should be discarded when the needle becomes dull, has been bent, or has come into contact with any surface other than the skin; if reuse is planned, the needle must be recapped after each use.

Syringe reuse may carry an increased risk of infection in some individuals. Patients with poor personal hygiene, an acute concurrent illness, open wounds on the hands, or decreased resistance to infection for any reason should not reuse a syringe. Patients should periodically inspect the skin around an injection site for unusual redness or signs of infection. Individuals should consult their physicians before initiating the practice of syringe reuse and whenever injection-site infection is suspected. Before syringe reuse is considered, it should be determined that the patient is capable of safely recapping a syringe.

The syringe being reused may be stored at room temperature. The potential benefits or risks, if any, of refrigerating the syringe in use or of using alcohol to cleanse the needle of a syringe are unknown. Cleansing the needle with alcohol may not be desirable, because it may remove the silicon coating that makes for less painful skin puncture (ADA, 1995).

It is important to warn patients who plan to reuse syringes against drawing alcohol up into a syringe to cleanse it. This practice has resulted in serious infections and necrosis when alcohol has been injected later accidentally.

Used syringes and needles should be discarded into a puncture-resistant disposal container. Local trash-disposal guidelines should be followed.

Complications of Insulin Therapy

Common complications of insulin therapy are as follows:

Hypoglycemia

The major complication of insulin therapy is hypoglycemia. Most patients who inject insulin have this problem at one time or another. If a patient injects too much insulin, exercises too much, does not eat enough or at the appropriate times, the blood glucose level can fall low enough to cause hypoglycemia or an "insulin reaction." Patients should be taught to monitor blood glucose levels, be alert for the signs and symptoms of hypoglycemia, and learn the appropriate measures to treat hypoglycemia (see chapter 7). Alcohol consumption should be limited as previously discussed, and alcohol should be drunk only with food to prevent a hypoglycemic episode.

Lipodystrophies

Lipodystrophies (atrophy and hypertrophy) can occur with insulin administration. Lipoatrophy, a pitting appearance of the subcutaneous tissue, is an immune reaction related to insulin source or purity that occurs in a small number of patients. The switch to a highly purified insulin will reduce the occurrence of atrophy. Injecting the highly purified insulin around and in the affected areas may also reduce the atrophied appearance. Lipohypertrophy is an area of subcutaneous tissue that is thickened and hard. It can be prevented by rotation of injection sites.

Effects of Chemicals and Medications

Certain chemicals and medications can affect blood glucose levels. Those that increase the levels include corticosteroids, estrogens, epinephrine, lithium, phenytoin, thyroid preparations, potassium-depleting diuretics, nicotinic acid in large doses, diazoxide, and large quantities of caffeine. Patients should also be alert for sugar added to medications, especially cold remedies or cough syrups.

Allergic Reactions

Allergies to insulin are not common, but they may occur. Both local reactions with rashes and cutaneous manifestations and systemic effects (serum sickness, anaphylaxis) may occur. Previously, because of less pure insulins, patients had allergic reactions more often. Zinc or protamine (used to prolong insulin action times), preservatives, and the vial stoppers have all been implicated as causes of local insulin reactions. Because of the increased purity of human insulin, changing from an animal insulin to human insulin is often effective in controlling the reactions. If reactions are systemic, desensitization may also be necessary.

Insulin Resistance

Insulin resistance is defined as the use of more than 200 units of insulin daily. This complication has been associated with a variety of conditions, including Cushing's syndrome, acromegaly, hemochromatosis, acanthosis nigricans, and morbid obesity. Use of U-500 insulin is indicated for these patients. Because of its greater concentration, the volume of insulin that must be injected is reduced.

Insulin Therapy Regimens

In people without diabetes, insulin and glucagon are released throughout the day. For blood glucose levels to be completely normal in patients with diabetes, it would be necessary to mimic this normal physiology. Thus, the best treatment would be a regimen of background or basal insulin with boluses of insulin before meals. Although many patients still take a single daily dose of insulin, diabetologists are clearly moving toward the use of multiple injections of human or highly purified pork insulin.

Dosing schedules *(Figure 4-1)* vary for patients with diabetes, depending on the amount of endogenous insulin secreted, the degree of insulin resistance, and the individualized goals of blood glucose management. In people without diabetes, the body produces approximately 25–40 units of insulin in 24 hr. If a person needs only 15–20 units of insulin to maintain glycemic control, it is obvious that endogenous insulin is being secreted.

The starting dose of insulin is usually based on the patient's weight: 0.5–1.0 units of insulin per kilogram of body weight per day. On the basis of the target established for blood glucose control, adjustments are made to achieve that goal. Self-monitoring of blood glucose is an essential component in adjusting the insulin timing and dosage. Patients differ in their response to insulin and also in their daily habits of diet, exercise, medications, and lifestyle. Therefore, many different insulin regimens are used.

Some patients are able to achieve control of diabetes with one injection a day. This dose is usually taken in the morning to improve blood glucose levels during the day. However, it is sometimes taken at bedtime to lower the fasting blood glucose level. With this regimen, an intermediate-acting insulin such as NPH or Lente is often used. Also used for this regimen is a combined dose of short- and intermediate-acting insulins or a premixed combination insulin. This regimen works best for patients who still secrete some insulin and is used for those with type 2 diabetes.

Two injections a day, one in the morning and one in the evening, are a common regimen. An intermediate-acting insulin may be injected twice daily, that is, once before breakfast and once before dinner or bedtime.

Another regimen is to use split doses of regular insulin with intermediate-acting insulin. This "split-mixed" regimen is considered conventional therapy. The total amount of insulin needed is usually given in a proportion of two-thirds of the insulin in the morning before breakfast and one-third before dinner.

Use of more injections of insulin a day is considered intensive therapy. This is used most often by patients who seek "tight" diabetes control and is generally more often used by those who have type 1 diabetes.

Three injections of insulin a day can be given in a variety of ways, depending on individual needs and lifestyle. A regimen that uses a split-mixed injection before breakfast, short-acting insulin before dinner, and an intermediate-insulin at bedtime often works well for patients who have a problem with elevated levels of blood glucose in the morning. Another regimen uses Ultralente insulin combined with regular insulin twice a day, before breakfast and dinner, and regular insulin

FIGURE 4-1 Time of action of insulin

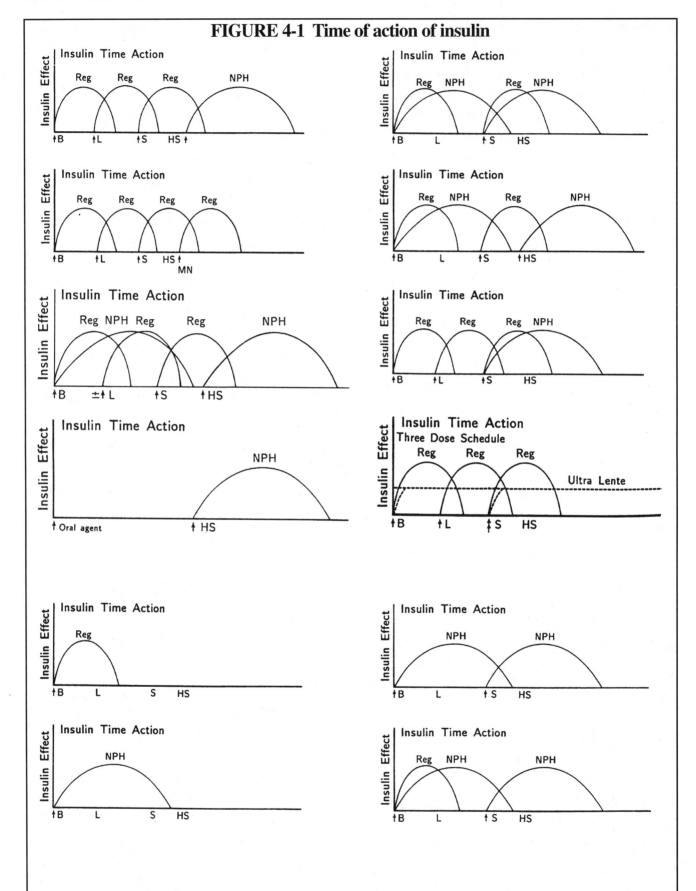

Source: American Association of Diabetes Educators. (1993). *Core curriculum for diabetes educators.* Wichita: University of Kansas, School of Medicine.

only before lunch. This regimen is useful in patients with an erratic lifestyle. A third method is to use regular insulin before breakfast and lunch and a split-mixed dose before dinner.

Some methods of intensive management use four injections a day. One frequently used regimen is referred to as "the poor man's pump" because of its similarity to the way insulin is delivered by the insulin pump. In this method, regular or rapid-acting insulin is injected before each meal, and intermediate or long-acting insulin (NPH, Lente, or Ultralente) is used at bedtime. The doses of regular or rapid-acting insulin are usually calculated before each meal and depend on the blood glucose level and the content of the meal to be eaten. The dosage of the longer acting insulin, which provides a steady background rate of insulin throughout the day, usually remains fixed. Occasionally four injections of regular insulin at about 6-hour intervals are used. This regimen is most often used in acute situations when blood glucose levels are out of control.

Insulin Adjustments

Insulin adjustments are made by each patient's physician with the increasing input of the patient. They are based on laboratory data, results of home blood glucose monitoring, and subjective information from the patient. As patients become increasingly knowledgeable about diabetes and their own bodies, many physicians encourage them to take a more active role in insulin adjustments. Often, with the proper instruction, patients can make dose adjustments independently.

Certain guidelines for adjustment are taught to these patients. The basic principle is to change the dose of insulin when blood glucose values are abnormal for 3 days in a row without any apparent cause (e.g., dietary indiscretion). The dosage should not be changed by more than 2 units at a time and should be kept at the new level for at least 3 days before further adjustment. Only one part of the regimen should be adjusted at a time to allow

the influence of the change on the total regimen to take effect. Knowledge of the action times of the various types of insulin is essential to dosage instruction. For example, if the blood glucose level is high before lunch, the regular or rapid-acting insulin taken before breakfast should be adjusted (increased), because this is the insulin with peak action at this time.

Injection Aids

If patients are squeamish about injecting themselves directly, several injection aids are available.

Automatic Injectors

With automatic injectors, the syringe is filled with insulin as usual and placed in the injector, which is spring loaded. After the area to be injected is selected and prepared, the injector is set against the skin, and the touch of a button forces the needle through the skin. The patient must then push the plunger of the syringe to inject the insulin.

Insuflon and Button Infusers

The Insuflon is a small teflon catheter that is inserted into the subcutaneous tissue and left in place for up to a week to allow multiple injections through a port without repeated punctures of the skin. Button infusers are similar to this device. Both are useful for patients who require multiple daily injections and who wish to avoid multiple punctures. However, in both cases, patients have the inconvenience of having a device constantly attached to the body.

Jet Injectors

Jet injectors are advertised as devices that require no needle for insulin administration. With a jet injector, air under intense pressure forces the insulin through the skin. The injection is not totally without sensation and may also cause bruising if improper pressures are used. Jet injectors are beneficial for patients who cannot tolerate the use of needles. Disadvantages of these devices include the cost, the inability to visualize the insulin in the injector, and the cleaning and maintenance of the device.

Insulin Pen

The insulin pen uses insulin dispensed in cartridges. Each cartridge contains 40–150 units of insulin. Needles are disposable and easily changed. This device, which looks like a fountain pen, is easily portable. The correct dose is dialed into the pen (audible clicks on some pens make then usable by patients with vision problems), and the needle is inserted and a plunger depressed to deliver the insulin. Prefilled and disposable pens are also available.

Injection Aids for Patients with Vision Problems

Several injection aids are available for patients with vision problems. Syringe magnifiers can help patients read dosage markings on the syringes. Insulin gauges and click-count syringes (clicks count out unit measures) are helpful in assuring correct dosage. Needle guides and vial stabilizers assist with inserting the needle into the vial. These devices can facilitate independence for a patient who has limited or no vision.

Insulin Pump Therapy

Insulin pump therapy is a method of intensive insulin management. Successful use of this method requires a high level of knowledge in diabetes management and a strong commitment on the part of the patient. This therapy requires frequent self-monitoring of blood glucose levels—at least four times a day—and meticulous care of the equipment.

The currently available pump therapy is known as continuous subcutaneous insulin infusion. It is an "open-loop" system. This term means that the amount of insulin is not automatically regulated by the user's blood glucose levels. Rather, a "link" is required to complete the feedback loop. The system requires the patient to monitor his or her blood level of glucose, determine the amount of insulin

needed, and program the pump to deliver the insulin. Only regular or rapid-acting insulin is used for this therapy. Velosulin BR® (buffered regular) Insulin is usually recommended for insulin pump use as it minimizes crystallization and blocking in the infusion line.

The pump is programmed to deliver a continuous basal amount of insulin throughout a 24-hour period that will take care of fluctuations in blood glucose levels when the patient is not eating. Before the patient eats a meal, the level of blood glucose is measured. On the basis of this reading, the target blood glucose level, and the content of the meal, a bolus amount of insulin is programmed into the pump and immediately delivered.

Many patients who use an insulin pump use carbohydrate counting to estimate the amount of insulin required for each meal. Advantages of pump therapy include a greater flexibility in meal timing and content and greatly improved control of blood glucose levels. Disadvantages include the danger of rapid development of diabetic ketoacidosis if the flow of insulin is interrupted, skin infections at the infusion site, and a "blunting" of hypoglycemic awareness.

Only one "closed-loop" system, the Biostator®, has been developed. With this machine, the patient's blood glucose levels are constantly monitored, and insulin is delivered in a continuous flow to meet the patient's needs. With this system, blood glucose can be maintained at target levels without the necessity for self-monitoring of the levels. Because it is the size of a television set, this system is not practical for home use.

GLUCAGON

Glucagon is a pancreatic hormone that plays an important role in maintaining glycemic levels by stimulating the liver to release glucose in response to low levels of blood glucose. Glucagon emergency kits are now available to be used as treatment for severe hypoglycemia. This product should be used for serious hypoglycemic reactions in which patients are unconscious and cannot take anything by mouth and emergency staff are not available to treat the reaction with an injection of 50% dextrose. In a health care setting, if hypoglycemia develops in a patient without an intravenous line, and the patient is unconscious, glucagon is used until venous access can be obtained. Glucagon is effective only if the patient has adequate hepatic glycogen (stored glucose in the liver) stores (See Chapter 7 discussion of hypoglycemia).

Glucagon is supplied as a dry powder in a vial with a prefilled syringe of diluent. Once the hormone is reconstituted, it should be used immediately. If not used at once, it can be stored at 41°F (5°C) for up to 48 hours. The dosage for adults and children more than 5 years of age is 1.0mg. Children less than 5 years of age should be given half of this amount. Glucagon can be injected either subcutaneously or intramuscularly, whichever is faster. Full onset of action occurs in 5–20 minutes (see chapter 7). If response to the treatment is inadequate another dose may be needed. A common side effect of glucagon administration is that nausea and vomiting may occur as the patient returns to consciousness.

EXAM QUESTIONS

CHAPTER 4
Questions 28–36

28. What is the appropriate action to take if vials of NPH insulin have sediment, clumping, or frosting of the bottle?

    a. Mix the insulin more thoroughly.

    b. Refrigerate the vials.

    c. Return the vials to the pharmacy.

    d. Use the insulin as usual.

29. What is the most common complication of insulin therapy?

    a. Lipodystrophy

    b. Urticaria

    c. Hypoglycemia

    d. Anaphylaxis

30. Which of the following statements about the use of glucagon is correct?

    a. It can be injected subcutaneously or intramuscularly.

    b. It should be mixed up and kept ready for use at all times.

    c. It should be injected whenever blood glucose levels are less than 60mg/dl.

    d. It should never be injected if the patient is unconscious.

31. When will a patient who takes 12 units of regular insulin and 25 units of NPH insulin at 7:30 a.m. have the first insulin peak?

    a. In 2–4 hours

    b. In 0.5–1 hours

    c. In 10–12 hours

    d. As soon as food is ingested

32. Under normal conditions, insulin is absorbed most rapidly from which of the following areas of the body?

    a. Abdomen

    b. Arm

    c. Leg

    d. Thigh

33. Which of the following is a mechanism of action of oral hypoglycemic agents?

    a. Increase the rate of carbohydrate metabolism

    b. Stimulates insulin secretion

    c. Increases the rate of glucose production by the liver

    d. Decreases the number of receptors on the cell surface

34. Which of the following statements about use of regular and NPH insulin mixed in the same syringe is correct?

    a. The injection should be administered within 1 minute after the insulins are mixed.

    b. The patient should administer the injection within 5 minutes after mixing the insulins or wait 24 hours before using the mixture.

    c. These two insulins should not be mixed in the same syringe.

    d. The injection can be premixed and refrigerated and is stable for one month.

35. Which of the following is a sulfonylurea?

    a. Metformin

    b. Glucotrol

    c. Prandin

    d. Glucophage

36. Liver function must be closely monitored with which of these oral antidiabetic agents?

    a. Glipizide®

    b. Orinase®

    c. Avandia®

    d. Amaryl®

CHAPTER 5

MONITORING DIABETES

CHAPTER OBJECTIVE

After completing this chapter, the reader will be able to discuss the various types of monitoring used in diabetes management, including indications for and values of each type.

LEARNING OBJECTIVES

After studying this chapter, the reader will be able to:

1. Recognize the advantages and disadvantages of various methods of blood glucose monitoring.

2. Recognize quality assurance issues related to blood glucose monitoring.

3. Recognize the advantages and disadvantages of various types of urine glucose testing.

4. Indicate the use of various types of monitoring in the management of diabetes.

INTRODUCTION

More than 100 years ago, the first laboratory tests for sugar in the urine were developed. Prior to that, diagnosis of diabetes was actually based on tasting the urine of the possibly diabetic person. In 1907, Stanley Benedict refined the copper-reduction test for use in home testing of urine. The test was known as Benedict's test and was much simpler and more convenient than the one done in the laboratory. It was the sole method of home testing for the next 35 years (Pollack, 1953).

In 1941, Ames Laboratories developed the Clinitest for testing urine. In this system, a tablet of reagent, a few drops of urine, and a few drops of water are placed in a test tube. The result is a chemical reaction that causes intense heat and "boiling." Many people severely burned their hands when using this method. By 1956, a dipstick method of monitoring had been developed.

All these tests for measuring glucose in the urine at home are semiquantitative, and thus the results are only a crude reflection of the quantities of glucose in the bloodstream. In addition, because urine is used for testing, the results are a reflection of what the actual blood glucose level was hours before the test, and it is impossible to detect hypoglycemia. The use of urine for testing was also aesthetically displeasing. Urine testing is still used today, although most often in tests for ketones.

In 1962, another revolution in diabetes care occurred. Keen and Knight showed that a drop of blood obtained by sticking the finger could be placed on a strip of filter paper and successfully analyzed in the laboratory. Thus was born home blood glucose monitoring. Today in 2 minutes or less, patients can find out what their blood glucose level is at the time of testing and make adjustments in medication, food, and exercise to regulate blood glucose levels. Thus, it is now possible to attain "tight" control of diabetes, with blood glucose levels consistently in or near the normal range. This advance in measuring blood glucose has placed the management and control of diabetes within the patient's own domain. Further developments include tests for glycohemoglobin and microalbuminuria to give more precise information about the long term control of diabetes.

GOALS OF MANAGEMENT

The reason for any testing in diabetes is to help the patient achieve better control of blood glucose levels. Therefore, goals for management should be established first. The goals will then guide the type and frequency of testing to be done. Acceptable goals for management of diabetes have been a topic of much discussion. The standards of control accepted by the ADA in 1999 *(Table 5-1)* consist of a range of types of control.

When the goals for diabetes control have been established, a monitoring program can be developed to determine treatment needs and evaluate the effectiveness of the treatment. Patients with diabetes are expected to be active participants in the process. They not only collect the data used but also make decisions about treatment.

URINE TESTING

Although the current trend in diabetes management is to use blood glucose testing, in some situations, urine testing is still appropriate. Until the 1960s, urine tests were extremely cumbersome and time-consuming. Now, several urine tests are available that are relatively inexpensive and more reliable than previous tests. They can be used to alert patients to potential hyperosmolar syndrome or ketoacidosis when diabetes is out of control.

TABLE 5-1
Diabetes Management Goals

Glucose Goals

- HbA1c 7% (average glucose of ≤150 mg/dl)
- Fasting glucose 80–120 mg/dl, bedtime glucose 100–140 mg/dl

Other Goals

- Blood Pressure 130/85 or lower
- HDL over 45 mg/dl
- LDL under 130 mg/dl or with Cardiovascular Disease under 100 mg/dl
- Triglycerides under 200 mg/dl

The Renal Threshold

The blood glucose level at which glucose will begin to spill into the urine is called the renal threshold *(Figure 5-1)*. In most persons, the average threshold is about 180–200 mg/dl. The threshold also increases with age. If a patient has a renal threshold of 200 mg/dl and his or her urine test is negative for glucose, the patient's blood glucose level has been less than 200 mg/dl in the period since he or she last urinated or voided. The test result does not, however, give any other information about the blood glucose levels.

If the same patient has a positive urine test, his or her concentration of blood glucose has been more than 200 mg/dl for some time prior to the time he or she last voided. As shown in *Figure 5-1,* the patient is spilling glucose into the urine sometime between 7 and 11 a.m. The test result does not indicate when the blood glucose level was high or if it is still high at the time of voiding. In this example, the blood glucose level is less than 120 mg/dl at 11 a.m. even though the level of glucose in the urine is high. When the patient voids a second time at about 11:30 a.m., the results of a urine test indicate that although blood glucose levels were high, they are now below the renal threshold. This find-

FIGURE 5-1

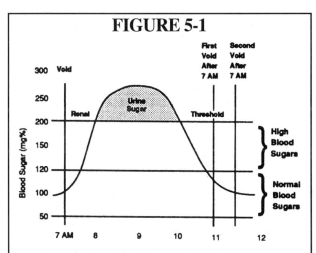

Spilling of glucose when blood levels exceed the renal threshold. Urine tests would be positive for glucose.

Source: Lodewick, P. (1988). *A diabetic doctor looks at diabetes: His and yours.* Waltham, MA: RMI Corporation.

ing illustrates why a second voiding of fresh urine may give a better idea of what the actual blood glucose level is at the time of voiding.

If urine testing is to be done, it is best to determine the patient's renal threshold by obtaining several plasma glucose levels and comparing the results with those of urine glucose tests. Both the method that will be used at home for testing and a laboratory analyzer should be used.

Urine Testing for Glucose

The position of the ADA on urine glucose testing is stated in the published clinical practice recommendations:

The basis for urine glucose measurements is the fact that glucosuria is roughly correlated with hyperglycemia. Urine testing is painless and less expensive than self-monitoring of blood glucose [SMBG]. However the use of urine glucose concentrations to estimate blood glucose concentrations in diabetes management is undesirable for the following reasons:

1. The renal threshold for glucose excretion in healthy adults corresponds to a plasma concentration of 10 mM (180 mg/dl). In many adults, particularly those with long-standing diabetes, this threshold may increase substantially. Thus, marked hyperglycemia may exist without glucosuria. Conversely, some individuals, particularly children and pregnant women, may have very low or variable renal thresholds, resulting in glucosuria with euglycemia. Urine glucose levels imprecisely represent blood glucose concentrations.

2. Fluid intake and urine concentrations can affect test results.

3. The test reflects an average level of blood glucose during the interval since the last voiding, and not the level at the time of the test.

4. A negative urine test does not distinguish between hypoglycemia, euglycemia, and mild or moderate hyperglycemia. Therefore, urine testing is of little help in achieving the management goal of avoiding hypoglycemia and hyperglycemia.

5. Urine testing, which involves comparing the color of the test strip against a printed chart, is less accurate than a digital readout of a blood glucose meter. It poses a problem for patients who are color blind or have other visual impairments.

6. Some drugs may interfere with urine glucose determinations (ADA, 1995).

For patients who cannot or will not perform SMBG, urine glucose testing can be considered an alternative that can provide useful, albeit limited, information. If patients choose to perform urine glucose testing, they should fully understand the test limitations (ADA, 1999).

Methods of Testing

Two methods are used for urine glucose testing: The glucose oxidase method provides semiquantitative indications of the amount of glucose present in the urine. Diastix, and Chemstrip uG are examples of this type of testing. The copper sulfate reduction method provides a more quantitative test. An example of this type is the Clinitest system.

Some of the available products measure both glucose and ketones in the urine.

Diastix® (Bayer Corporation). With the Diastix system, the test strip is dipped in a sample of urine for 2 seconds After 30 seconds, the color of the strip is compared with the color chart. The advantages of this test include its sensitivity and ease of use. In addition, the results are obtained quickly, and the colors are easy to read. Disadvantages include the following: It is the least accurate urine test (Olson, 1988). Vitamin C and aspirin can cause falsely low glucose readings, and ketones can affect the readings. The highest reading possible is only 2%. (Keto-Diastix® measures both ketones and glucose in the urine.)

Chemstrip uG® (Roche Diagnostics). With the Chemstrip uG system, the strip is dipped into a sample of urine for 1 second or less and then drawn along the rim of the container to remove excess urine. After 2 minutes, the color of the strip is compared with the color chart. This test system has several advantages. It offers a wide range of results, from $^1/_{10}$% to 5%. It is convenient, the colors are easy to read, and the results are accurate during pregnancy. Chemstrips are not affected by the presence of ketones in the urine and are useful for people with high or low renal thresholds. Disadvantages include difficulty in reading the color if the strips have been damaged by humidity. Also, large doses of vitamin C can cause false-negative readings. (Chemstrip uGK® reads both glucose and ketones.)

Clinitest® (Bayer Corporation). In the 5-drop Clinitest method, 5 drops of urine are mixed with 10 drops of water, and a Clinitest tablet is added to the mixture. A "boiling" reaction occurs. Fifteen seconds after the boiling stops, the tube is shaken, and the color of the contents is compared with the color chart. If the color of the solution passes through orange to dark green during boiling, the result is called a "pass-through" reaction, which indicates that the level of glucose is more than 2 g/dl. If a pass-through reaction occurs, the 2-drop method should be used, which can measure a higher glucose level. The procedure is the same as with the 5-drop method, except that only 2 drops of urine and a different color chart are used. The 2-drop method can measure glucose levels up to 5 g/dl. The main advantage of the Clinitest method is that it is the most accurate of urine glucose tests (Olson, 1988). In addition, the colors are easy to read, and damage of test tablets by humidity is easy to detect. The method has several disadvantages. The test kit is bulky, and the test is awkward to use. High doses of vitamin C, aspirin, and some antibiotics can cause false-positive results. The boiling mixture can cause burns. Finally, the system is less accurate than other methods of urine testing during pregnancy.

Twenty-four hour urine test. In the past, urine samples collected 24 hours apart were used to determine the average level of control over a 24-hour period. This type of test has been almost totally replaced by the glycohemoglobin test. Twenty-four hour urine tests are sometimes used now in children who have a poor growth pattern or in those who use urine testing for monitoring and have evidence of poor control despite negative urine tests.

Frequency of Testing

The frequency recommended for testing depends on the type of diabetes, the goals for management, and whether urine glucose testing is an adjunct to testing blood glucose or is the only testing done.

Patients who use self-monitoring of blood glucose on a regular basis probably have no reason to also use urine glucose testing. For patients who monitor blood glucose levels only two or three times a week and have a normal renal threshold, daily urine glucose testing can be an adjunct to monitor control. If urine glucose testing is the only means of monitoring, checking the urine at least once a day and varying the times of testing between fasting, 2 hours after meals, and at bedtime can give some indication of the level of control. Keeping written records in a diary will help provide the information necessary to interpret the meaning of this type of testing.

Urine Acetone or Ketone Testing

Ketones appear in the urine when fat has been used as a source of energy. Fats are metabolized when a person is on a weight-loss diet or is under-nourished and physical activity takes place. When calories are reduced, less insulin is secreted into the bloodstream by the pancreas in people who are nondiabetic and in patients who have type 2 diabetes. The low levels of insulin allow the body to use fat as an alternative source of energy, and a small amount of ketones is produced. In patients with type 1 diabetes, the presence of ketones in the urine with high blood glucose levels indicates a potentially dangerous lack of insulin.

Methods of Testing

Three methods are commonly utilized to determine the presence of ketones in the urine.

Acetest® (nitroprusside) tablets (Bayer Corporation). With the Acetest system, a drop of urine is placed on a nitroprusside tablet. After 30 seconds, the color of the tablet is compared with a color chart. If ketones are present, the color will range from lavender to deep purple. The results are read as negative, small, moderate, or large. The advantages of this method are that the reagent does not react with ß-hydroxybutyrate and that it can be used to

test blood and estimate ketonemia. Among the disadvantages, L-dopa and large amounts of phenylketones and sulfobromophthalein and phenolsulfonphthalein can cause false-positive results.

Ketostix® (Bayer Corporation). With the Ketostix system, the test strip is dipped into a sample of urine. After 15 seconds, the color of the strip is compared with a color chart. The colors and range are similar to those obtained with Acetest tablets, and the results are interpreted in a similar manner. An advantage of Ketostix strips is that they are wrapped in foil and keep for longer periods than other strips. Therefore, they are more likely than other strips to maintain potency if not used often. Keto-Diastix measures both ketones and glucose.

Chemstrip K® (Roche Diagnositics). With the Chemstrip K system, the test strip is dipped into a sample of urine. After 1 minute, the color of the strip is compared with a color chart. The colors and range are similar to those obtained with Acetest tablets and Ketostix strips, and the results are interpreted in a similar manner. Chemstrip uGK can be used to measure both ketones and glucose.

Recommendations for Testing for Ketones

In patients with type 1 diabetes, urinary ketones may be an indication of developing ketoacidosis, a medical emergency. Generally a ketone test should be done during acute illness or stress; when blood glucose levels are consistently 240 mg/dl or more or urinary glucose is more than 1%; or when any signs and symptoms of ketoacidosis such as nausea, vomiting, or abdominal pain occur (ADA, 1995). Testing for ketones in these circumstances is critically important in children.

Starvation ketosis may occur in pregnancy if the caloric or carbohydrate intake is low. Consequently, most pregnant women are asked to test the first morning voiding for ketones.

Patients with type 2 diabetes are not routinely taught to do ketone testing, because they are not ketosis prone. Some physicians require ketone testing for patients involved in weight-loss programs. When ketones are present and the blood glucose levels are normal, loss of weight in patients with type 2 diabetes is due to fat metabolism.

Ketonuria that occurs at other times is much less significant. After a hypoglycemic reaction, ketones may be present because of the "rebounding" of blood glucose. Ketones may also be found in the urine during a fever or in minor amounts during physical exertion, especially in extreme heat without adequate carbohydrate intake (Krall & Beasler, 1989).

KIDNEY FUNCTION TESTS

A major concern in patients with diabetes is the possible development of renal insufficiency. Physicians obtain measurements of serum creatinine and blood urea nitrogen levels to monitor kidney function (*Table 5-2*). An increase in the levels beyond normal indicates a rather late phase in loss of kidney function, when the damage is thought to be irreversible. The creatinine clearance test is a measure of the filtering capacity of the kidney, but it is not particularly effective in detecting the early stages of renal failure.

The early stages of diabetic kidney disease can be more easily detected by monitoring the excretion of protein in the urine. Normally, no protein is excreted in the urine. The presence of protein in the absence of signs and symptoms may indicate thickening of the microvasculature of the basement membrane, which allows protein leakage. Dipsticks can be used to measure the protein that has leaked into the urine. A positive result indicates the onset of glomerular dysfunction. Also a 24-hr urine collection can be done to assess the amount of protein creatinine present.

Recently, sensitive radioimmunoassays that detect minimal amounts of protein in the urine (microalbuminuria) have been developed. These dipstick tests are simple to perform and offer the opportunity to detect changes 5–10 years before the other tests would indicate problems. This early warning of microvascular changes allows changes in management that can result in the preservation of renal function. Products available include the Chemstrip Micral® (Roche Diagnostics), which can detect protein levels of 20 µg, and Albusticks® (Bayer Corporation).

BLOOD TESTING

Office, Clinic, or Hospital Methods

When a patient visits the office of a health care provider or a clinic or is hospitalized, laboratory methods used to assess diabetes control include assays of plasma levels of glucose and glycosylated hemoglobin. In addition, capillary glucose testing is done in all these settings. The oral glucose tolerance test is done much less often than before, but it is sometimes still used in the diagnosis of diabetes.

Plasma Glucose Testing

The results of plasma glucose testing give an indication of the degree of glucose control and insulinization at a particular time. When used in a physician's office or a clinic without home testing as the only indicator of diabetes control, the results are difficult to interpret. The major difficulty with this type of testing is that it is difficult to know what this one test may indicate. Blood glucose levels vary widely during the day. The test may have been done on a patient who became conscientious only on the day preceding the test, and therefore the results are not an indication of usual values. The patient may also be ill, causing an unusual increase in the level of blood glucose. Several other factors, including time of day, relationship to

---

TABLE 5-2
Typical Normal Ranges for Renal Function Tests

Test Name	Normal Range
Blood urea nitrogen (BUN)	7–25 mg/dl
Serum creatinine	0.7–1.4 mg/dl
Creatinine clearance	Over 100 mL/h
Urinary protein	0 mg

Source: Reprinted from Wylie-Rosett, J., Villeneuve, M. E., & Engel, S. S. (1987). Monitoring of comprehensive diabetes management. In M. Powers (Ed.), *Handbook of diabetes nutritional management* (p. 98) with permission of Aspen Publishers, Inc. © 1987.

---

insulin action, type of food eaten that day, exercise, and so forth, can influence the results and lead to erroneous impressions of blood glucose control. Because plasma glucose levels cannot adequately reflect the overall degree of glucose control, they should be supplemented with an assay for glycosylated hemoglobin (ADA, 1995).

Glycosylated Hemoglobin Assays

Glycohemoglobin was first discovered in the red blood cells by Samuel Rahbar in 1969. As a result of this discovery, a test that measures the percentages of glycosylated hemoglobin in the blood to indicate longer term diabetes control has been available since 1977. This test gives a value for the average level of glucose for the preceding 3 months.

After hemoglobin is produced in the body, it remains in the red blood cells for the entire life of the cells, approximately 120 days. Glucose molecules gradually attach to the hemoglobin molecule as they circulate in the bloodstream. The attachment (glycosylation) is irreversible and is not grossly affected by brief fluctuations in the blood glucose level. Because the hemoglobin molecule has a life span of 120 days, this test reflects the average blood glucose concentration over that period *(Table 5-3)*. Researchers have shown that the levels of glycohemoglobin are an excellent indicator of the level of control.

Two different tests are done, and it is important to know which one was done to correctly compare the results with the expected normal values. Tests for HbA1 measure the combination of all the fractions of the hemoglobin molecule: HbA1a, HbA1b, and HbA1c. Usual normal values for this test are 8–9%. Tests of HbA1c are a measure of the glycosylation of the c fraction only. The normal value for this test is usually 4–7%, because the test measures only one fraction.

Researchers are studying the feasibility of using tests for glycosylated hemoglobin rather than oral glucose tolerance test, which is currently the standard, for screening patients and diagnosing diabetes. Using tests for glycosylated hemoglobin has several advantages. The assay is a simple laboratory test that requires a small amount of blood. No fasting or special preparation is required. The information gained from the test is valuable in assessing overall control. The results can supplement those of blood glucose testing. High values warn the patient that changes in management are needed, and normal or close to normal values confirm that management is on track. One disadvantage is that blood glucose levels indicated by the glycohemoglobin value will appear to be normal if the glucose concentrations fluctuate widely (e.g., from hypoglycemic levels to sharp increases).

The ADA recommends that glycohemoglobin testing be done at least twice a year in patients who are meeting their treatment goals and more often (quarterly) for patients who are not meeting their glucose goals or who are changing treatment regimes.

This test is most often done in the physician's office with a venous blood sample. Kits are now available for performing this test at home and when used properly, these kits provide accurate results with only a fingerstick sample of blood. The sample is mailed to the kit supplier and the results are reported to both patient and physician.

TABLE 5-3
Correlation Between Mean Glucose Levels and Glycohemoglobin Values

Mean Glucose	Glycohemoglobin
<120	3.8–6.3 Normal
120–150	6.3–7.0
150–200	7.0–8.0
200–250	8.0–9.5
250–300	9.5–11.0
>300	>11.5

Source: Glycosylated hemoglobin. (1983). Calabasas Hills, CA: Endocrine Sciences (800 444-9111).

Glycosylated Albumin and Fructosamine Assays

Both albumin and fructosamine (ketoamine) become glycosylated and can be used to assess diabetes control. The life span of these substances is shorter than that of glycosylated hemoglobin, and therefore measurements of glycosylated albumin and fructosamine indicate the control for shorter periods (e.g., 1–3 weeks). These measurements are useful in pregnancy, when large swings of blood glucose must be avoided, and in patients with newly diagnosed diabetes in whom a short period of control must be evaluated.

Glucose Tolerance Testing

The oral glucose tolerance test is used in several different ways to test patients with disorders of glucose homeostasis. Several factors can affect the test results, and overdiagnosis can be a problem (Nelson, 1990).

Proper preparation of the patient before the test is important. This test should not be used for patients who are chronically malnourished or on bed rest. The patient should have ingested at least 150 grams of carbohydrate on a daily basis for 3 days before the test. No caffeine or nicotine is permitted before or during the test. The patient should

be otherwise healthy, ambulatory, and not on any medications that could affect glucose tolerance.

The test should be scheduled for the morning after the patient has fasted for 10–16 hours. The test dose of glucose for a nonpregnant adult is 75 grams (see chapter 6 for discussion of the use of this test in pregnant women and in children). Blood samples are obtained before the test begins and then 0.5, 1, and 2 hours after the patient takes the test dose. The results are interpreted according to criteria established by the ADA (see chapter 1).

Use of the glucose tolerance test should be limited to patients who have signs and symptoms of diabetes but have a fasting plasma glucose level of less than 140 mg/dl, pregnant patients who have a positive 1-hour screening test for diabetes during their 24th to 28th week of pregnancy, and patients who may have acromegaly. The test should not be used to diagnose reactive hypoglycemia (Nelson, 1990).

HOME BLOOD GLUCOSE MONITORING

The most important technological development in the treatment of diabetes since the discovery of insulin is blood glucose monitoring. Self-monitoring of blood glucose levels is also sometimes referred to as home blood glucose monitoring, capillary blood glucose testing, or self monitoring blood glucose (SMBG). Self-monitoring provides immediate information about current blood glucose levels and allows the patient to respond promptly with the appropriate treatment and to make decisions about medication, diet and exercise.

Self-testing has enabled caregivers and patients to fine-tune blood glucose control, troubleshoot problems on the spot, and safely institute intensive insulin management. "Normoglycemia" has become a realistic and attainable goal for patients with diabetes as a result of this testing (ADA,

1999). Countless hospital admissions have been avoided through this method of management, which allows accurate measurements of metabolic control in the home that can be used to make clinical decisions.

Two basic methods are used to monitor blood glucose levels. With the visual method, the changes of a reagent strip are compared with a chart. With blood glucose meters, the device reads the strip and gives a digital result. For accurate results, the patient must follow the proper method for obtaining a sample of capillary blood and the proper procedure for using the equipment.

Obtaining a Sample for Testing

The patient should be taught the easiest and least painful method of obtaining a small drop of blood. Using the side of the finger at the outer edges at the ends of the fingers is recommended. The sides of the finger have fewer nerve endings than other parts of the finger and less contact with hard surfaces, factors that reduce tenderness in the area after testing. Puncturing the finger tip causes more discomfort. Ear lobes and toes can be used also. However, for patients with poor circulation in the lower extremities, use of the toes is not recommended.

Several kinds of automatic lancing devices are available (e.g., Soft Touch®, Penlet®, Unistix®, Autoclix®), and aid in shielding the needle from view and in controlling the depth of puncture. The drop of blood obtained must be large enough to cover the reagent pad to ensure accuracy.

Instructions for obtaining a capillary blood sample are as follows:

1. Clean the fingertip (warm water increases blood flow). Alcohol may be used but tends to dry the skin. If alcohol is used, be sure the finger is dry before the skin is punctured.

2. Stabilize the finger by resting it on a flat surface.

3. Place the lancing device on the side of the finger near the tip. Use minimal pressure to minimize the depth of penetration. Depress the button on the device to puncture the skin.

4. Hold the finger in a dependent position, and gently milk the finger to obtain a drop of blood.

Patients' skills in monitoring should be evaluated periodically (at least annually) to ensure accuracy. Results obtained by the patient should be compared with the results of a concurrent laboratory test for plasma glucose.

Methods of Monitoring

Visual Methods

There are several products currently available for use in visual testing. The range of blood glucose readings is from 20–800 mg/dl for some of the products. One advantage of visual testing is that a meter does not have to be purchased. The disadvantages are that the readings are only an approximation (e.g., between 180 and 240 rather than an absolute number); the accuracy of readings is dependent on color vision; and a small error in technique can cause substantial error in the results.

Blood Glucose Meters

Meters read blood glucose concentrations in the range of 20 to 600 mg/dl. Caution is advised in the readings at the extreme ends of the range. All the monitors provide fast results, usually in less than two minutes. Today's meters weigh less than a pound and run on batteries so they are very portable.

Two different technologies are used in glucose meters. Reflectance meters shine a beam of light onto a chemically treated test strip that has been stained with a drop of blood. The meter measures the amount of light the stain reflects and translates that into a blood glucose concentration in milligrams per deciliter. The paler the stain is on the strip, the lower the blood glucose reading is and vice versa. Biosensor or sensor meters convert a chemical reaction into an electrical charge that is caused by the reaction of glucose and the enzyme on the test strip.

In addition there is a difference in the calibration of the meters. Some meters reference whole blood and some reference plasma. Laboratory equipment references plasma. Laboratory values will be about 15% higher than readings from a meter which references whole blood. If patients are using a meter that references whole blood they will be surprised that their HbA1c readings are higher than they expected based on their meter readings. People with diabetes may use different meters during the day, but this becomes dangerous if one references plasma and the other whole blood. The differences in readings could lead to incorrect insulin doses.

Most of the meters sold today have a memory feature that will store 10–250 test results. This feature is a valuable tool for health care professionals to use during a visit to assess patients' monitoring. It is preferable for patients to actually keep a record book or diary of the blood glucose levels rather than relying solely on the meter's memory. Some units can also download the stored information into a personal computer as part of a data management system.

Monitors for Patients with Visual Impairments

Patients with severe visual impairments can be independent in performing self blood glucose monitoring. There are several blood glucose monitors on the market that give verbal instructions to guide a person through the entire testing procedure and give verbal test results. One monitor also provides an opening to place insulin bottles for identification so that patients can distinguish between short and long acting insulins to avoid errors in administration.

Recommendations for Use of Blood Glucose Monitoring

Anyone who has diabetes can benefit from self-monitoring of blood glucose levels. The ADA (1995) strongly urges self-monitoring for the following:

- Patients who are using insulin pumps or are taking multiple daily insulin injections with the goal of tight blood glucose control.
- Women who are pregnant or planning pregnancy.
- Patients using insulin who often have hypoglycemia and have problems recognizing the warning signs and symptoms.

In addition, the ADA recommends that health professionals encourage the use of self-monitoring for the following patients:

- Those who require insulin.
- Those whose renal thresholds are unusually high or low.
- Those who have unstable diabetes.
- Those who are trying to improve control.

Accuracy and Reliability of Blood Glucose Monitoring

Some of the monitoring systems are highly dependent on the skill of the operator; others are almost foolproof. The usefulness of the results, however, depends on the system's accuracy. Several factors can decrease the accuracy of the readings:

- Insufficient amount of blood placed on the strip.
- Inaccurate timing and incorrect wiping technique.
- Dirty optic window, which scatters light transmission.
- Variations in temperature and humidity (e.g., leaving the monitor or the test strips in a hot car trunk).

- Incorrect calibration of the meter.

- Defective or outdated strips.

- Hematocrits that are very high or low.

- Severe hypoglycemia or hyperglycemia.

- Hypotension, hypoxia, and elevated blood levels of triglycerides.

It is crucial that patients who use self-monitoring receive the proper training and have a clear understanding of how the results of monitoring are to be used in their diabetes care. Periodic comparisons should be made between results obtained by the patient' self-monitoring system and a fasting blood sample obtained at the same time and measured by a referenced laboratory (ADA, 1999).

Patients should also be taught correct procedures for using the quality control solutions provided for their individual system and the correct calibration and cleaning procedures. If a caregiver is doing blood glucose testing for the patient, proper handling of the blood sample, including using gloves to prevent transmission of blood-borne pathogens, must be taught.

Advantages and Disadvantages of Self-Monitoring

Several of the advantages of self-monitoring of blood glucose levels have already been mentioned. When used correctly, self-monitoring is an accurate and reliable system that provides immediate feedback and allows prompt reactions to variations in blood glucose concentrations. It is easy to use; the equipment is lightweight and portable. Patients who have difficulty with colors or limited vision can use digital readings or audio prompting.

Self-monitoring allows flexibility in lifestyle and gives patients a sense of control. Patients report satisfaction from their ability to participate fully in their care. Self-monitoring also serves as a concrete educational tool by providing feedback on the impact of diet, exercise, and medication on blood glucose levels. It is a tool for day-to-day decision

making and a reliable assistive device in the case of an emergency.

One of the biggest disadvantages and impediments to self-monitoring of blood glucose levels is the cost of strips and supplies. It has been estimated that the cost of performing four tests per day for 1 year is approximately $750. This amount is indeed minimal compared with the expense of hospitalizations, but for patients without insurance coverage, it is an overwhelming burden.

For some patients, pricking the finger is also a definite disadvantage. Particularly older patients may feel overwhelmed by the "machinery." As previously mentioned, the monitors are not reliable for extremes of hematocrit and blood glucose concentrations that are very high or very low, and in these cases, laboratory methods must be used.

Choosing and Using a Blood Glucose Monitoring System

Several factors should be considered before choosing a system for monitoring blood glucose. If cost is a consideration and vision is not a problem, visual monitoring may be the right method if exact readings of blood glucose values are not needed for insulin adjustments. The cost of monitors has decreased significantly and meters provide a simple method of determining exact readings of blood glucose values. Various features such as download capabilities or memory features appeal to individual consumers.

The goals of monitoring are paramount when deciding which monitor best suits a particular patient. Ideally, patients should try several systems before selecting one. If a patient is not comfortable with a system and later does not use it, money has been wasted, and diabetes care has not been well served.

It must be remembered that obtaining the blood sugar reading is only one aspect of care. A definite schedule for monitoring must be set up as well as a plan for data collection in the form of a diary and a plan for the use of the blood glucose data. Patients often do not know why they are checking their blood glucose level and often report that their health care providers do not review the diaries with them. General guidelines for when to check blood glucose levels include checking at the times when the information will be used to make decisions about treatment (e.g., at peaks of insulin times, to check postprandial changes in blood glucose concentrations, fasting levels) and in illness and emergency situations (e.g., when blood glucose levels are fluctuating or elevated). Patients often stop testing when they are asked to check very frequently (e.g., four times a day) and cannot understand why such frequent tests are needed.

The ADA (1999) recommends that the results of self-monitoring of blood glucose levels be used by health care providers to do the following:

1. Set glycemic controls.

2. Develop recommendations for pharmacologic therapy.

3. Evaluate the effectiveness of pharmacologic therapy.

4. Instruct patients on how to interpret and respond to blood glucose patterns.

5. Evaluate the effect of dietary factors on glycemic control.

6. Modify therapy during acute or intercurrent illness or when patients receive medications that affect glycemic control.

7. Modify the management plan in response to changes in activity.

8. Detect hypoglycemic unawareness and determine strategies for treatment.

DIABETES MANAGEMENT AND GUIDELINES FOR CARE

The frequency and timing of glucose monitoring should be dictated by the needs and goals of the individual patient. For most patients with type 1 diabetes the ADA recommends three to four tests daily. For patients with type 2 diabetes testing should be adequate to reach glucose goals. The DCCT and the UKPS Studies (see chapter 11) conclusively demonstrated that maintaining blood sugars in ranges of normal, or close to, normal blood sugars can reduce microvascular complications of diabetes. In order for patients to assess their range of blood sugars testing fasting blood sugars and two hours after their largest meal is recommended. This can be compared to HbA1c test results *(See Table 5-3)*. Blood glucose values under 120 mg/dl are considered excellent. A range of blood sugars over 200 mg/dl is considered poor control. The American Diabetes Association (1999) has specified a standard of care to be followed by all primary care providers when taking care of patients with diabetes *(Table 5-4)*.

Bedside Capillary Glucose Monitoring in the Hospital Setting

Nonlaboratory hospital personnel who perform bedside capillary glucose monitoring are subject to several regulations by the Joint Commission on Accreditation of Health-Care Organizations and other regulatory agencies. There must be adequate and documented training and periodic verification of competency of the personnel who do the testing. Hospitals must have written policies and procedures about the use of the test and quality control standards. Daily quality control tests must be done, and patients' records must include documentation that correlates with the quality control testing. In addition, procedures for the handling of the blood drop specimen must be consistent with the Occupational Safety and Health Administration

---

TABLE 5-4
American Diabetes Association
Diabetes Care Guidelines

Every primary care giver visit

• Blood Pressure check

• Foot Inspection

• Review goals for glucose, diet and exercise

Laboratory

• HbA1c two or more times per year

• Cholesterol, HDL, LDL, Triglycerides yearly

• Microalbumin yearly

Other Interventions

• Annual dialated eye exam

• Annual influenza vaccination

• Regular dental visits

• Diabetes education

---

guidelines for prevention of transmission of blood-borne pathogens.

Procedures must be specific about the protocols to use in laboratory verification of hypoglycemia and hyperglycemia. The position statement (ADA, 1986) by experts in the diabetes field elaborates on this topic:

In any instance where the result of a bedside glucose measurement may make a critical difference in the management of a patient with a life-threatening illness, the result must be confirmed by a hospital laboratory glucose determination. Also, caution should be exercised in the interpretation of bedside monitoring results in patients with severe anemia or polycythemia.

Comparison Hospital Bedside Monitoring and Laboratory Tests

The bedside glucose monitoring system in use in the hospital may use whole blood, which includes red blood cells. Laboratory assays generally use serum or plasma, which does not include these cells. Therefore, the results of assays of serum or plasma are usually 10–15% higher than the results of assays of whole blood (Bernstein, 1981). In addition, most laboratories analyze samples of venous rather than capillary blood, and after fasting or in a postprandial state, the amount of glucose in venous blood is generally 5 mg/dl lower than the amount in capillary or arterial blood (Bernstein, 1981). For example, for a patient who has been fasting, the blood glucose concentration is 200 mg/dl by laboratory tests (plasma, serum, or venous blood) and 175 mg/dl by self-monitoring (fingerstick and whole blood from a capillary). This is within the accepted range: laboratory value (200 mg/dl) - 15% = 200 - 30 = 170 mg/dl, and 170 + 5 = 175 mg/dl.

EXAM QUESTIONS

CHAPTER 5
Questions 37–45

37. To help prevent transmission of blood-borne pathogens, persons performing capillary glucose monitoring on another person should use which of the following?

    a. Face masks

    b. Reflectance meters

    c. Alcohol swabs

    d. Gloves

38. Which of the following is a necessary element of a quality assurance program for use of glucose meters in a health care facility?

    a. Memory capability

    b. Local calibration

    c. User training

    d. Comparison with glycosylated hemoglobin

39. Which of the following is a major advantage of glucose meters?

    a. Accurate at all hematocrit levels

    b. Wide range of values the meter reads

    c. Cost of meter and strips

    d. Ability of meter to diagnose diabetes

40. Which of the following tests should be done to evaluate impending ketoacidosis at home?

    a. Blood test for ketones

    b. Blood test for glucose

    c. Urine test for ketones

    d. Urine test for glucose

41. Which of the following is a major advantage of blood glucose testing over urine glucose testing?

    a. The results do not depend on the patient's renal threshold.

    b. The test is less time-consuming to perform.

    c. The procedure is easier to teach.

    d. The cost of the test is less.

42. Which of the following diagnostic studies is the most valuable in assessing a patient's long-term management of diabetes?

    a. Two-hour postprandial glucose test

    b. Six-hour glucose tolerance test

    c. Assay for glycosylated hemoglobin

    d. Assay for glycosylated nucleotides

43. The visual method of self-monitoring of blood glucose levels requires patients to do which of the following?

    a. Use a large amount of blood to obtain accurate results.

    b. Use a special color-coded meter.

    c. Wear special color-filtering glasses.

    d. Compare the color of a reagent strip with a color chart.

44. Which of the following can affect the accuracy of blood glucose readings?

    a. Microalbuminuria

    b. Elevated hematocrit

    c. High cholesterol

    d. High blood pressure

45. Which of the following tests reflects a patient's average blood glucose levels over a 2- to 3-month period?

    a. Protein electrophoresis

    b. Assay for glycosylated hemoglobin

    c. Assay for glycosylated lipoprotein

    d. Hemoglobin electrophoresis

CHAPTER 6

SPECIAL ISSUES IN MANAGEMENT OF DIABETES

CHAPTER OBJECTIVE

After completing this chapter, the reader will be able to discuss the special needs of patients with diabetes during specific life stressors (e.g., traveling, surgery) and able to describe interventions to meet these needs.

LEARNING OBJECTIVES

After studying this chapter, the reader will be able to

1. Specify self-care challenges that face elderly patients in managing diabetes.

2. Indicate special management concerns while traveling for patients with diabetes.

3. Specify the specialized techniques used to manage diabetes as a child matures.

4. List the surgical risk factors related to patients with diabetes.

5. Indicate four clinical implications for management of a pregnant woman who has diabetes or in whom the disorder developed during pregnancy.

6. Specify three risk factors for a poor clinical outcome in a pregnancy complicated by diabetes.

7. Recognize the specific guidelines for management of diabetes during pregnancy.

INTRODUCTION

The care of patients with diabetes presents particular challenges throughout the patients' life span, during times of stress such as surgery, and when the usual routine is altered by travel. This chapter provides information that health care providers can use to help patients cope with these special issues in diabetes management.

DIABETES IN THE ELDERLY

The care of older patients who have diabetes includes special considerations. The changes brought about throughout the life span add to the demands necessary to caring for a chronic condition. Goals for glycemic control are generally less stringent to allow for maximal life enjoyment and safety. An individualized plan of management is of paramount importance, because age in years is not an absolute indication of aging or loss of functional ability. People are definitely living not only longer but healthier lives today.

Diabetes is an important health problem among the elderly. Among those older than 65 years, more than 40% have diabetes (Funnell et al., 1998). It is estimated that in the year 2020, more than 50 million people will be over the age of 65. These figures clearly show that the number of older patients who have diabetes is ever increasing.

Aging and Barriers to Health Care

Many changes that occur as the life span lengthens produce impediments for health care. Normal physiologic changes associated with aging are often compounded by the concomitant presence of one or more chronic illnesses. Poor dexterity, decreased physical strength, and failing vision can make using equipment such as syringes and monitoring equipment difficult. Memory impairment and hearing loss can interfere with understanding directions and carrying out instructions. Loss of a spouse, changes in living arrangements, physical and emotional isolation, and decreased financial resources can severely affect a person's ability to function effectively in self-care requirements.

Four stages of advancing age and the problems that accompany the stages have been listed by gerontologists (Reichel, 1995):

1. 50–65 years, late adulthood or preretirement years. Health problems such as cardiovascular disease, diabetes, and arthritis begin to emerge.

2. 65–74 years, a time of change in lifestyle and social networks brought about by retirement, decreased income, and death of spouses and friends. During these years, health problems may become chronic.

3. 75–84 years, the beginning of "old age." Health, social, and financial problems threaten independent living.

4. 85 years and older, a time when independent living becomes difficult.

It is also crucial to remember that aging occurs at a different rate for each person. Although many 80-year-olds may find it difficult to walk a block or two, some are still doing marathon walking.

Effects of Aging on Glucose Tolerance

Rapid onset of type 1 diabetes in the elderly is unusual. Most older people with diabetes have type 2 diabetes. As all humans become older, glucose tolerance decreases. This change is particularly evi-

dent in postprandial blood glucose levels, which may increase by as much as 8–20 mg/dl with each decade (Lipson, 1985). Several possible hypotheses may account for the hyperglycemia that occurs with aging (Lipson, 1985):

- Decreased insulin secretion from beta cells

- Insulin resistance at the receptor sites, at postreceptor sites, or intracellularly

- Changes in body composition such as increased adipose tissue and loss of lean body mass

- Decreased physical activity

- Decreased peripheral glucose utilization

- Changes in diet

- The prevalence of coexisting illnesses and use of various drugs that contribute to hyperglycemia

Management Goals

Elderly patients with diabetes have several short-term risks for complications. High levels of blood glucose with glucosuria and weight loss predispose patients to acute illness and infections. Patients in this age group who have long-term poor control are particularly vulnerable to hyperosmolar hyperglycemic nonketotic syndrome, which has a high mortality rate (see chapter 7).

Many patients who have type 2 diabetes may have had asymptomatic hyperglycemia for some time before they sought medical care. This condition puts them at particular risk for many of the long-term complications of diabetes, such as stroke and renal insufficiency & amputation. Elderly patients who successfully managed their diabetes when they were younger may only need to modify management to accommodate the changes that accompany aging.

If diabetes is first diagnosed when a patient is elderly, several factors should be considered in establishing goals and a management program

(Table 6-1). An overriding principle should be to impose the minimum number of restrictions necessary and limit the number of life changes in establishing a realistic plan. Achieving normal or near-normal blood glucose levels may be a reasonable goal in a "young-old" person who has no other medical problems or complications. Maintaining normal blood glucose levels may be an unrealistic goal for an elderly patient with several other impairments and may contribute to hypoglycemia, which is a definite risk factor in this population. Hypoglycemia may contribute to confusion or result in unconsciousness, which could be mistaken for a transient ischemic attack or a cerebrovascular accident.

Include family members who are involved in daily care in all educational and clinical visits. Once treatment goals have been established, a management plan for diet, exercise, and medications should be made.

Diet

Nutritional interventions should avoid rigid or complex meal plans. For elderly patients who are overweight, even a modest weight loss often will substantially improve blood glucose control and minimize or eliminate the need for medication or insulin. This outcome can greatly simplify management for the patient. The elderly have many barriers to changes in food intake, including long-standing eating patterns, cultural traditions, physical impairments to food preparation, and financial constraints that dictate the types of food consumed. The help of an experienced dietitian and the patient's family members can be valuable in promoting optimal nutritional therapy. Consideration should also be given to supplementation with vitamins, minerals, and protein (Powers, 1987).

Exercise

A well-planned exercise program can greatly improve glucose tolerance in older patients. In

---

TABLE 6-1
Important Factors to Consider for Diabetes Management in the Elderly

Patient's remaining life expectancy

Patient's commitment

Availability of support services

Economic issues

Medical disorders

    Psychiatric disorder

    Cognitive disorder

    Diabetes complication

Major limitation of diabetes functional status

Source: Reprinted with permission from Lebovitz, H. (Ed.). (1991). *Therapy for Diabetes Mellitus and related disorders* (p. 157). Copyright © 1991 by the American Diabetes Association, Inc.

---

addition to dietary management, exercise can often be used for the management of diabetes in this age group. The intensity and type of exercise are of particular concern because of the high incidence of silent coronary disease in these patients and the risks of infection associated with injury. For the elderly, an exercise stress test and electrocardiographic evaluation are mandatory before an exercise program is prescribed.

Medications

If the treatment goals are not achieved with diet and exercise, antidiabetes agents are used. The most significant risk in using these drugs in the elderly is hypoglycemia due to renal or hepatic insufficiency. The use of longer acting agents is a particular problem because of the length of time the agents remain in the system; this persistence can produce prolonged hypoglycemia. For this reason, chlorpropamide (Diabinese®) is not recommended for use in the elderly (Lebovitz, 1991). It is also important to consider potential interactions of the oral antidiabetes agents and other drugs, because many older patients are taking multiple medications.

If oral medications are insufficient to establish control, insulin is used. The simplest regimen should be considered, such as a combination of oral medications with insulin at bedtime and or use of premixed insulins (one injection if possible). Again, hypoglycemia is the major concern and complication of therapy *(Table 6-2)*. The skills necessary for administration of insulin and monitoring (e.g., adequate vision, fine motor control, and cognitive function) must be carefully evaluated to be sure that the patient or the patient's caregiver is able to monitor blood glucose levels and administer the insulin safely.

Monitoring

It is generally agreed (ADA, 1999) that because of the high renal threshold in older patients, urine glucose tests are not helpful in management. As with other aspects of care, simplicity and ease without sacrificing safe care should be the principles guiding the type and frequency of monitoring. If a patient is following a fixed regimen, checking the blood glucose level before breakfast can provide a safety check in regard to nighttime low blood glucose levels or dangerous increases. When a patient is ill or the concentration of blood glucose remains elevated, more frequent monitoring will be needed. Assays of glycosylated hemoglobin at visits to the patient's physician provide an overall indication of the effectiveness of treatment.

SURGERY IN PATIENTS WITH DIABETES

According to estimates, patients with diabetes have a 50% chance of having surgery during their lifetime (Alberti, 1990). In the past, surgery in patients with diabetes was associated with an increased mortality rate. Now, with improved techniques and methods of

---

> ### TABLE 6-2
> ### Risk Factors for Hypoglycemia in Older Patients with Diabetes
>
> Impaired autonomic nervous system function
>
> Impaired counterregulatory responses
>
> Poor or irregular nutrition
>
> Cognitive disorder
>
> Use of alcohol or other sedating agents
>
> Polypharmacy
>
> Kidney or liver failure
>
> *Source:* Reprinted with permission from Lebovitz, H. (Ed.). (1991). *Therapy for Diabetes Mellitus and related disorders* (p. 160). Copyright © 1991 by the American Diabetes Association, Inc.

management, the risks have been reduced. However, the metabolic abnormalities and the complications associated with diabetes not only cause an increased risk of morbidity and mortality related to surgery but also are often the reasons that surgery must be done.

Management during the surgical period is complicated by both the metabolic abnormalities associated with diabetes and the presence of atherosclerotic disease, nephropathy, and autonomic neuropathy. Patients with diabetes also have an increase in the risk for postoperative infection (Arauz-Pacheco & Raskin, 1991).

The general management goals for surgical patients who have diabetes are to prevent hypoglycemia and ketoacidosis, to control hyperglycemia, to maintain normal electrolyte and fluid balance, and to resume oral feedings as soon as possible. An understanding of the physiology involved in the response to the stress of surgery is needed to provide this management.

Physiologic Changes During Surgery

Surgery has a profound metabolic effect on the body. The levels of counterregulatory hormones in the bloodstream increase. The sympathetic nervous system releases large amounts of epinephrine and norepinephrine (the catecholamines). This release causes an increase in the heart rate, which in turn causes an increase in blood pressure and dilation of the bronchi to increase the oxygen supply to the tissues. Blood is shunted to the vital organs in the body core along with the essential oxygen.

The release of epinephrine decreases the uptake of glucose by muscle tissue and inhibits the release of insulin from the pancreas. The catecholamines cause the glycogen stores in the liver to be broken down into glucose (glycogenolysis) and released into the bloodstream to supply energy needs. The glucocorticoids that are secreted stimulate the liver to supply additional glucose from protein conversion (gluconeogenesis). Glucose uptake by fatty tissues is inhibited by the glucocorticoids. In addition, breakdown of fats (lipolysis) occurs, increasing the serum level of fatty acids.

In patients without diabetes, the result of these metabolic changes during surgery is often an increase in the concentration of blood glucose into the range of 150–200 mg/dl. In patients with diabetes in whom insulin secretion is impaired, severe hyperglycemia with or without ketosis can occur unless replacement of insulin is adequate (Arauz-Pacheco & Raskin, 1991). Because patients fast before surgery, administration of insulin will cause hypoglycemia unless carbohydrates are also supplied. The degree of difficulty in managing patients depends on the extent and duration of the surgery.

Surgical Risk Factors

A number of metabolic and hemodynamic stresses can compromise the cardiovascular system and lead to myocardial infarction or congestive heart failure. Agents used in anesthesia can depress the function of heart muscle and may induce dysrhythmias. Events during surgery, including bleeding, can add to stress on the myocardium and may result in hypovolemia, hypotension, tachycardia, bradycardia, volume overload, fever, and shivering.

The risk of postoperative myocardial infarction is higher in patients with diabetes than in those without, and the infarction often is asymptomatic and causes no pain.

Nephropathy can make fluid management a concern, and it contributes to electrolyte abnormalities. Autonomic neuropathy can cause severe hypotension, especially during the induction of anesthesia. Increased rates of infection are associated with decreased effectiveness of leukocytes because of hyperglycemia. The risk for clotting and thrombosis is also increased.

Preoperative Management

For all elective surgery, preoperative care should include a thorough history and physical examination. Coronary artery disease and hypertensive vascular disease are common in patients with diabetes. Therefore, a complete evaluation of the patient's cardiovascular status, including special attention to orthostatic changes in blood pressure and changes in heart rate with respiration, should be done (Arauz-Pacheco & Raskin, 1991). Use of ß-blockers to control hypertension may increase the risks of hypoglycemia. Patients should also be evaluated for the risk of thrombosis and should receive anticoagulant therapy postoperatively if necessary. Concentrations of blood urea nitrogen, serum creatinine, electrolytes, and urine protein should be measured to evaluate renal function.

Orthostatic hypotension, neurogenic bladder, hyperesthesia or hypoesthesia, and gastroparesis are all diabetic neuropathies that can complicate the recovery from surgery. Physical assessment, including measuring blood pressure both when the patient is lying down and when standing, reflex and pin-prick testing, and determination of residual urine, should be done before surgery. Gastroparesis (see chapter 8) is more difficult to assess but may be suspected when a carefully kept record of blood glucose levels is available and indicates fluctuating blood glucose levels.

Control of blood glucose levels should be evaluated, and if needed, changes should be made to improve the concentration of blood glucose before elective surgery is scheduled. According to Alberti (1990), a preoperative goal is to maintain fasting blood glucose levels of less than 125 mg/dl and postprandial levels of less than 180 mg/dl. Chronically high blood glucose levels in patients result in dehydration, which must be corrected. Assays for glycosylated hemoglobin provide information about the overall status of blood glucose control for the 3 months before the test, and assays for glycosylated fructosaminc can help determine a more recent level of glucose control.

Intraoperative Management

It is important to remember that although patients with type 2 diabetes do have metabolic abnormalities of blood glucose control, they are still able to secrete insulin in response to hyperglycemia. In contrast, patients with type 1 diabetes do not secrete insulin and depend entirely on exogenous (external) supplementation of insulin. Therefore, insulin must always be given to patients who have type 1 diabetes.

It is ideal to keep glucose levels at or near normal at all times. However, maintaining these levels is difficult and increases the risk for hypoglycemia, which must be avoided. It is generally considered safer to err on the side of mild hyperglycemia. Thus, the goal is a blood glucose level of 125–200 mg/dl during surgery (Arauz-Pacheco & Raskin, 1991). Surgery should be scheduled early in the day to avoid prolonged fasting.

Several methods of insulin administration are used. Subcutaneous injection of insulin is associated with unpredictable absorption and variable glucose levels and usually is not used for major surgical procedures. Most of the regimens for major surgery include intravenous administration of regular or short-acting insulin and 5–10% glucose.

Glucose and insulin may be given in the same infusion mixture. The advantage of this method is that if the glucose infusion is stopped (e.g., disconnected or obstructed), the insulin infusion is stopped also, thus avoiding the risk of hypoglycemia. The disadvantage is that the method does not allow flexibility to change the delivery rate of either insulin or glucose to make adjustments for variations in blood glucose levels. Probably the best method is to administer insulin and glucose in separate infusions through the same vein (e.g., piggyback the infusions). This allows changes to be made in each infusion independently to respond to changes in glucose levels.

Electrolytes, especially potassium (necessary for glucose to enter cells), are also administered as needed. In patients with fluid restrictions or fluid overload, it may be necessary to administer dextrose in more concentrated forms (e.g., D50 through a central line) and to provide carbohydrates without large amounts of fluid. Blood glucose levels should be monitored hourly to maintain glucose levels in the desired range. Patients with type 2 diabetes who are using oral hypoglycemic agents or diet only to control their blood glucose levels may temporarily require insulin both intraoperatively and postoperatively. Only human insulin should be used to reduce the risk of sensitizing the patient.

For patients with type 2 diabetes who are undergoing fasting and minor procedures (e.g., local anesthesia, radiologic studies), the insulin or oral agent is usually stopped before the surgery and started again afterward. Because of their long half-life, long-acting oral agents should be discontinued at least 36 hours and preferably 72 hours before surgery. For patients with type 1 diabetes, either the morning dose of longer acting insulin is reduced (e.g., one half to two thirds of intermediate-acting insulin with no regular insulin) or a sliding-scale regimen of regular insulin is used during the perioperative period.

Postoperative Care

Infusion of glucose and insulin is continued until the patient's metabolic condition stabilizes. It is important to remember that for patients with type 1 diabetes, subcutaneous insulin must be started before the intravenous insulin is discontinued (see chapter 7) to avoid rebound hyperglycemia. The goal of postoperative care related to diabetes is to maintain blood glucose levels within a range that will promote healing, decrease the risk of infection, prevent the acute complications of hyperglycemia and hypoglycemia, and promote a sense of well-being.

Hyperglycemia can lead to ketoacidosis and electrolyte imbalances. Careful monitoring of glucose and electrolyte levels is important. Alterations in the electrocardiogram or rhythm strips or in the level of potassium (see chapter 7 for a detailed discussion of potassium shifts) may indicate a silent myocardial infarction. Adequate pain management is important, because pain can cause the release of counterregulatory hormones and increase the amount of glucose in the bloodstream.

Hypoglycemia may be difficult to detect in patients who are still recovering from anesthesia or are in pain and receiving narcotics. A decrease in blood pressure, an increase in the pulse rate, and irritability may be signs of hypoglycemia. The levels of blood glucose and the need for insulin may decrease dramatically as the stress of surgery diminishes or an infection subsides. If hypoglycemia is suspected, monitoring should be done immediately. Low concentrations of blood glucose require prompt intervention: ingestion of carbohydrates or an infusion of dextrose if the patient is not allowed anything by mouth (hospital protocols should be followed).

The surgical wound should be carefully observed for any signs of inflammatory changes or drainage. Impaired granulocyte function due to hyperglycemia can predispose patients to bacterial infections. Poor circulation due to microangiopathy can also contribute to postoperative infection. An increase in body temperature can be an indication of infection.

Careful monitoring of blood urea nitrogen and serum creatinine levels help in detecting acute kidney failure that may occur, especially after procedures with iodinated contrast agents. If these agents are used, the patient must be well hydrated before and after the procedure. Failure to void may be the result of a neurogenic bladder and may require treatment.

Total parenteral nutrition may be required in the postoperative period. Use of total parenteral nutrition can present special problems for patients with diabetes, because glucose is usually added to the feeding solution. The level of blood glucose should be monitored frequently, and the patient may require additional sliding-scale insulin to maintain blood glucose control. The doses of insulin needed during total parenteral nutrition are usually high. Often more than 100 units of insulin is required (Arauz-Pacheco & Raskin, 1991).

Returning to the normal meal plan as soon as possible will promote healing and reestablish homeostasis. At least 150–200 grams of carbohydrate should be given daily to prevent hypoglycemia and ketosis due to starvation (Powers, 1996). Problems with gastroparesis may complicate the recovery period. Signs and symptoms include gas, belching, a bloated feeling after meals, and a low blood glucose level after meals.

TRAVEL AND DIABETES

At one time, patients with diabetes were advised not to travel. The concern was that changing routines could upset the already complex and tenuous balance that had been established and that unfamiliar surroundings could spell disaster. This belief has changed. People with diabetes can travel anywhere in the world, but proper planning and preparation are essential.

Preparing for the Trip

Before planning a trip, patients should establish good diabetes management and blood glucose control. It is best to obtain any needed inoculations or vaccinations well in advance so that any reactions that could affect blood glucose levels will be over before the date of travel.

The names and addresses of English-speaking physicians at each destination will be helpful in case medical assistance is needed. For travel abroad, the address of the embassy or consulate at each destination will also be helpful. Medical insurance coverage in other countries is also important. Patients should check their insurance policies and obtain additional coverage if necessary. Policies are often available through travel agencies.

Packing

For patients with diabetes, eating the right foods and eating on time are essential. Travelers should always carry a supply of carbohydrate to treat reactions due to low blood glucose levels. A supply of supplemental food or a "food kit" is useful in case food is not readily available. Depending on the distance and length of travel, an emergency food kit may include the following: canned vegetable juice, canned fruit juice, dried fruit, crackers, cereal, peanut butter, canned meat or fish, cheese spread, nuts, Lifesavers, hard candies, and glucose tablets or gel. The kit should be readily available in hand or carry-on baggage.

Equipment for measuring blood glucose levels, ketone strips, insulin or oral hypoglycemic agents, alcohol swabs, cotton, and syringes should be kept in hand-carried luggage and not placed in checked baggage, which could be delayed or lost. Patients should take along two to three times the amount of supplies that will be needed during the trip to allow for breakage, spillage, or loss. An extra battery for

the glucose meter, a backup extra meter, and strips that can be read visually arc also useful.

Other items to pack include the following:

- A sun-blocking agent. Because many patients with diabetes heal poorly, they need to prevent sunburn-induced infections.

- A first-aid kit with moleskin to be used to prevent blisters on the feet and possible serious foot problems.

- Two pairs of properly fitting, comfortable walking shoes that can be worn alternately to prevent foot problems.

- A glucagon emergency kit to be used in case of severe insulin reactions. It can also be used to prevent low blood glucose if nausea and vomiting make eating impossible.

- Medication for nausea, vomiting, and diarrhea.

Travelers should wear a Medic-Alert® bracelet or similar type of identification. Prescriptions for insulin, medications, and syringes should be obtained before the trip. In addition, patients should have a handwritten and signed letter from their physician stating that they have diabetes and listing all current medications by brand and generic names.

For patients who use insulin who will be traveling in a foreign country, the letter should include the information about the need for syringes. This document will be important to reassure customs officials that the supplies are medical necessities. For the same reason, all medications should be left in their original and labeled containers. In addition, these patients should find out how insulin is supplied in the country they will be visiting and should become familiar with how to use insulin in different strengths (e.g., usually U-40 or U-80).

The Day of Travel

If a long trip by car is planned, it is wise for patients to have a snack before starting out. Stops should be scheduled to allow for determining blood glucose levels, taking medication or insulin, and eating appropriate meals and snacks. When a patient with diabetes sits for long periods, the concentration of blood glucose tends to increase, and circulation becomes sluggish. Periodic stops to take a walk and do some stretching exercises can help with both of these problems. Insulin should never be kept in a glove compartment or in the trunk of a car where it could become overheated. If the ambient temperature is high, the insulin is best kept in a cooler.

U.S. airlines usually can provide "diabetic meals." Provision for such meals must be arranged before the day of travel. It is not usually possible to arrange for diabetic meals on airlines in other countries. In these instances, taking a supply of appropriate food on board the airplane to supplement meals and provide snacks in case of delays is the best plan.

Patients who use insulin may need to make some adjustments in the insulin dosage when long flights are involved. The major concern of occasional travelers who have diabetes is to avoid hypoglycemia on the day of travel. It is not likely that hyperglycemia will occur as long as a reasonable dose of insulin is taken. Slightly elevated blood glucose levels on the day of travel are not a concern and are certainly preferable to hypoglycemic episodes.

Several algorithms are used to adjust insulin doses. In general, when patients are traveling east and time is lost, insulin doses are decreased. For example, in traveling from Boston to Paris, 6 hours are lost, which is one fourth of a day. In this case, the dose of insulin could then be reduced by one fourth. When patients travel an equal distance west, the reverse of this rule would be followed. Another method is to switch from longer acting insulins to sliding-scale regular insulin until arrival and then establish a routine on the new time with the normal dosage. The most important guidelines are to estab-

lish a plan for managing diabetes during travel by consulting a physician or health professional before the scheduled trip, to check blood glucose levels frequently, and to carry supplemental food to eat if low blood glucose levels occur.

DIABETES IN CHILDREN AND ADOLESCENTS

Diabetes in childhood and adolescence develops for the same reasons as it does at other stages in life (see chapter 1). In type 1, the most common form in children, the child is probably born with a genetic predisposition to diabetes. Antibodies to islet cells are present in the bloodstream at diagnosis. These antibodies indicate active destruction of the beta cells in the pancreas. The factors that trigger the destruction are not known for certain but may include coxsackie virus B4, mumps virus, and Epstein-Barr virus (the cause of infectious mononucleosis). Children who were infected with rubella virus (German measles) before birth (congenital rubella syndrome) also have a greater risk of diabetes developing in late adolescence (Krall & Beaser, 1989). Type 1 diabetes occurs in children and adolescents at a rate of 13.8 to 16.9 per 100,000 for Caucasian American children and from 3.3 to 11.8 per 100,000 for African American children (Tull, 1995). Approximately 100,000 children and adolescents have diabetes. The worldwide incidence of type 1 diabetes varies with the highest incidence in Sweden, Finland and Norway and the lowest incidence in Japan.

The months of January through April are a peak season for the diagnosis of diabetes. It is postulated that this seasonal peak may occur because infections in the cold and flu season unmask the preexisting decrease in beta cell function and provide the stress that tips the balance into diabetes.

Diagnostic criteria for children and adolescents are generally the same as those for adults. Oral glucose tolerance testing is not recommended in children.

Types of Diabetes

Diabetes in children or adolescents is almost always type 1. Consequently, type 1 diabetes was called juvenile diabetes, childhood diabetes, or brittle diabetes until it became known that the disorder is not limited to children. Type 1 diabetes can develop at any age, although it is rare in infancy. The most common age for the onset is 10–12 years, and boys and girls are equally affected.

Type 2 diabetes does sometimes occur in children. These children are usually grossly overweight and often have a family history of diabetes. The usual signs and symptoms at the time of diagnosis are much less pronounced and do not include ketoacidosis. This type of diabetes is often most responsive to weight loss.

A rare form of type 2 diabetes known as maturity onset diabetes of the young (MODY) is inherited in an autosomal dominant fashion. That is, it occurs in three or more generations, one parent transmits the disease, and approximately one half of the members of each generation are affected. This disease occurs most often in Asian Indians and black Americans and is often diagnosed early in adolescence. It can often be treated with oral antidiabetic agents. Secondary causes of diabetes in children and adolescents include cystic fibrosis, use of high doses of steroids or antileukemic drugs, and pancreatectomy.

Diabetes at birth or within the first 6 weeks of life is exceedingly uncommon and usually occurs in low-birth-weight infants who are premature or small for gestational age. This syndrome is known as transient neonatal diabetes. Most infants recover within 2 months.

Onset and Stages of Development

The development of diabetes has four stages (Krall & Beaser, 1989).

Acute Onset

In adults, the development of type 1 diabetes is sometimes slow. In children, the signs and symptoms usually begin rapidly, especially the tremendous thirst, frequent urination, and profound loss of weight. The recurrence of bed-wetting is often a clue that something has happened. The child typically eats well, perhaps even more than usual, but loses weight and energy and becomes listless, weak, and irritable.

Additional signs and symptoms include blurring of vision, deterioration of school performance, headaches, chest and abdominal pain, diarrhea or constipation, and headaches. These can rapidly progress to dehydration and ketoacidosis (Kussmal's respirations, fruity breath odor, nausea, vomiting, alterations in level of consciousness). The initial signs and symptoms may be confused with those of the flu or infection with a stomach virus.

Blood glucose values are usually in the range of 300–1,000 mg/dl and make the diagnosis clear. If the diabetes is detected in the early stages, the pancreas is still able to produce some insulin, but not enough to keep blood glucose at normal levels. In this situation, the child may require only one injection of insulin a day.

Remission or Honeymoon Stage

A period of reduced need of insulin occurs in about 50–60% of patients. The patients appear to improve, and their own insulin is enough to keep blood glucose levels in control. The reason for this return of function is not completely understood. One theory is that a decrease in inflammation and edema surrounding the beta cells allows the cells to function again.

In most patients, this remission lasts only a short time (3–6 months). This period often raises false hopes that the diagnosis was a mistake or that the diabetes went away. Because the remission is short, it is generally considered best not to completely discontinue insulin during this time but to continue small doses to avoid false hopes.

Intensification Phase

The remission phase often ends after an infection or other acute illness or with increased growth or the onset of puberty. During the third stage, the intensification phase, the amount of insulin secreted by the pancreas fluctuates, and maintaining blood glucose control is difficult, because of the variations in the amount of injected insulin needed.

Total Diabetes

In the final stage, insulin is no longer produced, and the patient is totally dependent on the availability of injected insulin. Fluctuations in the need for insulin continue because of factors such as physical growth and growth spurts, puberty, hormonal factors, and variations in activity levels and food intake.

Treatment

The overall goal of treatment of children and adolescents with diabetes is to help patients control the diabetes so that their daily function is equivalent to that of their peers. The specific goals are as follows:

- Relieve the signs and symptoms of hyperglycemia

- Prevent acute complications such as ketoacidosis and hypoglycemia

- Ensure normal growth, development, and maturation

- Reduce the risks of long-term complications

- Achieve optimum psycho social development

- Promote well-being and vigor

There has been no consensus on blood glucose goals for pediatric practice. Target ranges for blood glucose depends on the judgement of the health care provider and goals of the child and their family. Guidelines for target levels range from 80–120 mg/dl for fasting and 80–180 mg/dl at other times of the day. For children less than 6 years of age the target range begins at 90 mg/dl and the upper level is 200 mg/dl (Funnell et al., 1998).

Initiation of Treatment

Children with newly diagnosed type 1 diabetes are usually admitted to the hospital for 3–5 days for initiation of treatment and education on basic diabetes management. Quite often the children are ill and require intensive management. The diagnosis of diabetes in a child is a major shock and crisis for the child's family, and time and a safe place for the process of healing and adjustment to begin are needed.

Monitoring

In order to achieve the goals stated, good control of blood glucose and keeping the concentration as close to normal levels as possible, is necessary (ADA, 1999). Home blood glucose testing is the preferred method of monitoring and is done two to five times a day. Children and their parents are taught to use patterns of glucose levels to make adjustments in insulin dosages. Goals for control of blood glucose levels vary with the age of the child. The goals are more liberal for young children than for those of school age or older.

Because of the immature neurologic system of young children, every effort must be made to avoid severe hypoglycemia, which could cause permanent damage. For infants and young children, fingers, toes, and heels are used for glucose testing.

Assays for glycosylated hemoglobin are particularly useful in children and adolescents, in whom blood glucose levels tend to fluctuate a great deal. The HbA1c value serves as a report card and can be used as a goal to achieve when assays are done every 3–4 months. Testing for ketones during periods of illness or persistently elevated blood glucose levels is also especially important in this age group, because they are so prone to the sudden development of ketoacidosis.

Insulin

The insulin requirements are calculated on the basis of body weight. Approximately 0.5-1.0 units of insulin per kilogram is needed. During growth spurts, when high levels of growth hormone cause elevations in glucose levels, the need for insulin may increase to 1.5–2.0 units/kg. Calories will also need to be increased at this time. The Mauriac syndrome is a manifestation of long-term poor glucose control due to underinsulinization. It is characterized by growth retardation, sexual infantilism with delayed puberty, hyperlipidemia, a round face, a protuberant abdomen, and hepatomegaly.

Infants and very small children with diabetes usually require very small amounts of insulin. It is difficult to measure parts of a unit accurately even with low-dose syringes. Parents are instructed to use a solution available from the insulin manufacturer to dilute U-100 insulin to the strength of U-50 or even U-25 insulin. Diluting the insulin makes the measurement of fractions of a dose easier (e.g., 2 units of U-25 insulin = 0.5 units of U-100 insulin).

Nutrition

Nutrition counseling for children with type 1 diabetes and their parents requires careful instruction and frequent reinforcement. The success of the nutritional program depends on individualization and flexibility. The material is best taught by a dietitian who is experienced in working with children. In general, a child of average weight needs 1,000 calories/day at age 1 year and an additional 100 calories/day for each additional year up to the onset of puberty. Caloric requirements change rapidly in the growth years and may reach levels as high as 3,000 calories/day in adolescent boys.

Coordinating meals with the time and action of insulin injections is important. The results of blood glucose monitoring can be used to evaluate the results of deviations from the food plan and help in making adjustments.

Anorexia nervosa, bulimia, or a combination of the two is an ever-increasing problem. Treatment of type 1 diabetes that is complicated by an eating disorder is difficult. A purging behavior unique to patients with type 1 diabetes occurs with self-induced glycosuria due to overeating and taking inadequate amounts of insulin, which also results in weight loss. These special situations require intensive and specialized management.

Exercise

During childhood and adolescence, exercise is usually spontaneous. Active participation in organized sports has positive implications for children with diabetes and should be encouraged. However, aerobic endurance exercise is preferable to activities that involve straining and increases in systemic blood pressure (e.g., weight lifting). Monitoring the concentration of blood glucose, eating snacks before exercising, and carrying a supply of readily available glucose can ensure safe and enjoyable exercise.

Education

Learning survival skills is the first goal in the educational process. Parents and children should be taught the general plan and goals of treatment and how to achieve the goals. The division of responsibility for diabetes care between the child and the child's parents is first a function of the child's age and developmental stage and second a function of the individual personalities involved. In general, the child should be encouraged to take as much responsibility for self-care as possible. An excellent way for children to learn diabetes management is to attend a diabetes camp, where diabetes education is a vital and integral part of the program.

The most important skills needed for diabetes management are the following:

1. Insulin injection technique and simple dose adjustments

2. Prevention and treatment of insulin reactions

3. Self-monitoring of blood glucose levels and relating levels to insulin dosages

4. Diet fundamentals

5. Sick-day rules

Even a relatively minor illness, such as an upper respiratory tract infection, can quickly upset the metabolic balance of children with type 1 diabetes and may lead to diabetic ketoacidosis. Therefore, learning sick-day management skills (see chapter 8) is of major importance.

It is most important to help children and adolescents with diabetes lead lives that are as full and active as those of their peers. Management of diabetes should not dominate their lives. Critical elements of the plan of care should include support systems that facilitate these goals.

DIABETES AND PREGNANCY

The treatment of pregnant women who have diabetes has been one of the greatest successes in the history of diabetes care. Pregnancy for women with diabetes was once a severe threat to the health and well-being of both mother and baby. Until fairly recently, women with type 1 diabetes were counseled by their physicians to avoid the risks of pregnancy, to adopt children instead. The picture today is quite different.

Diabetes Mellitus is one of the most commonly occurring complications of pregnancy, affecting more than 150,000 pregnancies in the US annually. In medical centers that specialize in the management of diabetes during pregnancy, the perinatal mortality figures for offspring of insulin-dependent diabetic women approach the 1.6–2.0% of the general population. This success is achieved only through ideal care and a concerted effort to normalize maternal metabolism throughout gestation. Such care is provided by a team of diabetes and perinatal experts and requires the full cooperation of the patient and her family.

Normal Metabolism in Pregnancy

During pregnancy, the fetus is totally dependent on the mother for an uninterrupted supply of nourishment. For the pregnant woman to provide this supply of nourishment, several adaptations in metabolism must occur. During the early months of pregnancy, maternal fat storage occurs (anabolism). During this first half of pregnancy, "accelerated starvation" can occur if food is withheld. In this situation, concentrations of free fatty acids and ketones reach higher levels in pregnant women than in nonpregnant women.

Normally, insulin inhibits the production of ketones. During pregnancy, however, secretion of human placental lactogen and other counterregulatory hormones antagonizes the effects of insulin. This state of insulin resistance may be responsible for the diabetogenic effect of pregnancy (Schwartz, 1991). Ketosis has been associated with IQ changes in the fetus. Plasma levels of glucose and amino acids also decrease more markedly in pregnant women who are fasting than in nonpregnant women. During the late stages of pregnancy, the woman's insulin levels are higher than in the nonpregnant state, and the ingestion of food results in a twofold to threefold increase in insulin secretion (Coustan, 1991).

This state of maternal hyperinsulinemia and insulin resistance is characteristic of normal pregnancy *(Figure 6-1)*. In the late stages of pregnancy, the progression of nighttime fasting ketosis is so pronounced that delaying breakfast can result in significant ketonuria.

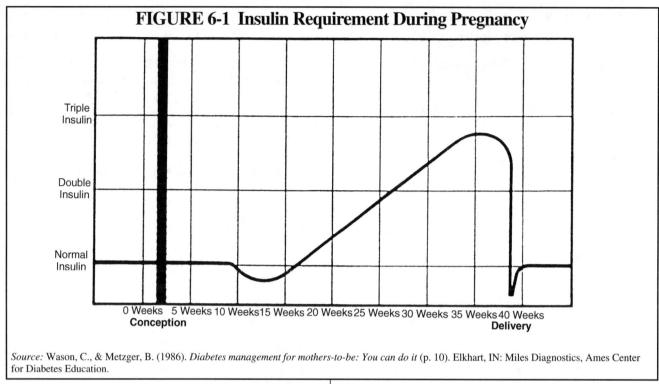

FIGURE 6-1 Insulin Requirement During Pregnancy

Source: Wason, C., & Metzger, B. (1986). *Diabetes management for mothers-to-be: You can do it* (p. 10). Elkhart, IN: Miles Diagnostics, Ames Center for Diabetes Education.

Ingestion of food results in higher and more prolonged increases in blood glucose levels in pregnant women than in nonpregnant women (Coustan, 1991). Because of this high and prolonged increase in blood glucose after meals, transplacental delivery of glucose to the fetus occurs, which promotes fetal growth.

Metabolism in Pregnancy Complicated by Diabetes

The adaptations that occur in the early stages of pregnancy are minimal, but if food intolerances develop or hyperemesis occurs, the adaptations can complicate the management of diabetes. Insulin antagonism results in maternal hyperglycemia, which in turn causes an increase in the concentration of blood glucose in the fetus. In addition, larger amounts of maternal amino acids and other fuels cross the placenta to the fetus. These larger amounts cause the fetus to secrete high levels of insulin (fetal hyperinsulinemia), resulting in growth of insulin-dependent organs (e.g., liver), fat and increased abdominal girth. This combination of fetal overnutrition and hyperinsulinemia con-

tributes to the morbidity and mortality of infants of diabetic mothers.

Neonatal Complications

Several risks to the infant are increased in a pregnancy complicated by diabetes. The rate of major congenital anomalies in a nondiabetic pregnancy is approximately 1–3%. This increases to 6–8% in pregnancies in which type 1 diabetes is poorly controlled. Caudal regression and cardiac, renal, and central nervous system anomalies are the most common types of defects found in the infants of diabetic mothers. Good control of maternal blood glucose levels in the first trimester of pregnancy when organogenesis occurs can decrease the incidence of these defects.

When diabetes is not well controlled during pregnancy, the developing fetus receives more glucose, protein, and fatty fuels than are required for normal growth and development. Because insulin from the mother does not cross the placental barrier, the fetus secretes additional insulin to use the large amounts of glucose and other fuels it receives.

At the time of delivery, when the blood supply from the mother is discontinued, the baby continues to produce excess amounts of insulin, which may result in neonatal hypoglycemia. The exact blood glucose level that is considered hypoglycemic in infants is a matter of controversy, although many clinicians accept that levels less than 40 mg/dl indicate hypoglycemia (Strand & Ehrenkranz, 1991).

The increased secretion of insulin by the infant in response to excessive delivery of glucose and other fuels from the mother may result in macrosomatia. This disorder is manifested by increased fetal growth of adipose tissue, muscle, and liver. Macrosomatia can result in a difficult childbirth because of the position of the shoulders of the fetus and in injury and asphyxia at the time of birth. Stillbirth is now a rare complication of delivery when diabetes is well controlled before and during delivery, and sophisticated methods of fetal monitoring are used.

Nowadays, respiratory distress syndrome does not often occur in infants of diabetic mothers. In the past, obstetricians preferred to deliver infants of diabetic mothers as early as 3–4 weeks before the due date to prevent stillbirth. The result of this practice was that respiratory distress syndrome sometimes occurred because of the immaturity of the lungs of the neonate. Infants of women with diabetes can have delayed lung maturation and inhibition of surfactant production (Strand & Ehrenkranz, 1991). As a result of the improved ability to ensure good diabetes control, advances in the sophistication of fetal monitoring, and the ability to assess fetal lung maturity, the incidence of this complication has been reduced.

Hyperbilirubinemia, hypocalcemia, polycythemia, and renal vein thrombosis are additional complications that occur more often in the infants of diabetic mothers than in those of nondiabetic mothers. Infants should be carefully assessed for the signs of these complications. When promptly initiated, treatment is usually effective.

Maternal Risk Factors

The system used most often to assess the risk factors in pregnancy in women with diabetes is the White Classification System *(Table 6-3)*. This system, which includes seven categories or classes of risk, was developed by Priscilla White. It uses the woman's age at the onset of diabetes, the duration of the diabetes, and the presence of vascular complications to predict the outcome of pregnancy. In the system developed by Pederson and Molsted-Pederson (1965), classification is based on five prognostically bad signs of pregnancy that they associated with poor outcomes in diabetes and pregnancy: ketoacidosis, pyelonephritis, pregnancy-induced hypertension, poor clinic attendance, and self-neglect by the mother.

Although both these systems help detect patients at risk for poor outcomes, the most important predictors of the outcome of pregnancy are the degree of metabolic control achieved, the presence of diabetic vascular complications, and the signs defined by Pederson and Molsted-Pederson. These factors appear to be more important than the age of onset or the duration of diabetes in the mother (Buchanan, Unterman & Metzger, 1985).

Approximately 0.2–0.3% of all pregnancies occur in women with insulin-treated (type 1 and type 2) diabetes (Connell, Vadheim & Emanuel, 1985). The incidence of gestational diabetes is approximately 2–3%.

Preconception Care and Counseling for Women with Diabetes

In order to ensure the best possible outcomes for pregnancy and diabetes in women who are diabetic, care should begin before conception. All diabetic women of childbearing age should receive counseling about the potential risks of an unplanned pregnancy. Women who have diabetes

---

TABLE 6-3
White Classification

A classification system for diabetes and pregnancy developed by Priscilla White. This system has been used as a predictor of pregnancy outcome. It is based on age at onset of diabetes and the presence or absence of vascular disease.

G = Carbohydrate intolerance diagnosed during pregnancy. It is the same as the NDDG classification for gestational Diabetes Mellitus (GDM).

A = Class A: Glucose intolerance diagnosed before pregnancy.

B = Class B: Disease that began at age 20 or later or that has been present for 9 or fewer years with no vascular disease.

C = Class C: Disease that began between the ages of 10–19 years or that has been present for 10–19 years with no vascular disease.

D = Class D: Disease that began before age 10 or that has been present for 20 or more years or with vascular disease such as background retinopathy or calcified iliac or femoral arteries.

F = Class F: Disease complicated by diabetic retinopathy.

H = Class H: Diabetes complicated by cardiovascular disease.

R = Class R: Diabetes complicated by proliferative retinopathy.

Source: California Diabetes and Pregnancy Program. *Guidelines for care* (p. 207).

---

should follow a preconception protocol before they stop using contraception.

Any woman with diabetes who is planning pregnancy should have a thorough assessment for any vascular complications, with particular emphasis on retinopathy and nephropathy. Mild background or treated proliferative retinopathy is not an absolute contraindication to pregnancy. However, worsening of severe background or proliferative retinopathy can occur in pregnancy (Coustan, 1991). It is not clear whether this worsening is due to the pregnancy, the natural progression of the retinopathy, or the abrupt institution of improved diabetic control. This problem is best treated by photocoagulation (laser therapy) before and during pregnancy.

Diabetic nephropathy is one of the most critical complications that affects the outcome of pregnancy and is the leading cause of death in diabetic

patients less than 40 years old. The risks of preterm labor, stillbirth, neonatal death, and fetal distress are significantly increased in pregnant diabetic women who have this complication (Reece & Quintero, 1991).

Coronary artery disease occurs more commonly at a younger age and is more severe in patients with diabetes than in patients without. Women with known coronary artery disease are usually counseled not to attempt pregnancy. Patients with uncontrolled hypertension are also usually advised to avoid pregnancy (Reece & Quintero, 1991).

Use of oral antidiabetes agents during pregnancy is contraindicated because these agents cross the placental barrier. Women with type 2 diabetes who use these drugs are counseled to discontinue using them and to use insulin if necessary for blood glucose control.

Planning of the pregnancy is extremely important to ensure an optimal outcome. Use of birth control pills may cause increases in the concentration of blood glucose unless an adjustment in insulin is made. Establishment of excellent blood glucose control for at least 6 weeks before conception is recommended. This practice will ensure normal blood glucose levels in the first trimester and help reduce congenital anomalies during organogenesis. Assays for glycosylated hemoglobin or fructosamine are used to document normalization of blood sugars.

Management During Pregnancy

Normal blood glucose levels are lower in pregnant women than in nonpregnant adults. The goals for pregnant women with diabetes are to normalize blood glucose to those levels throughout the pregnancy. The target levels are fasting and premeal blood glucose concentrations of 70–90 mg/dl and postprandial concentrations that are less than 140 mg/dl one hour after meals and less than 120 mg/dl two hours after meals (Jovanovic-Peterson, 1994). Blood glucose levels are monitored frequently, often as many as four to five times a day.

Urine testing for ketones is done on the first morning urine specimen and anytime the blood glucose level is more than 150 mg/dl. The presence of ketones in the urine in the morning after an overnight fast is evidence of starvation ketosis, which can be prevented by increasing dietary intake in the evening. If ketones are present when blood sugar levels are elevated, ketoacidosis may be developing, and immediate medical care is needed.

Medications, such as terbutaline, (used to treat premature labor), often cause increases in blood glucose levels. Frequent assays for glycosylated hemoglobin are commonly used during pregnancy to monitor overall blood glucose control.

Nutrition

Adequate calories are needed to provide for weight gain in underweight and normal weight women and for weight maintenance or minimum weight gain in obese women. Usually 100–300 additional calories are needed in the second and third trimester. Weight gain should be controlled with 25–35 pounds recommended for normal weight women. Recommended weight gain is usually 1 lb/week during the second or third trimester. Weight loss is contraindicated. The dietary composition is the same as recommended for nonpregnant adults. Three meals a day with two to three snacks are usually recommended. Pregnant women require an additional 10 grams protein per day, 1200 mg/day of calcium, 400 ug/day of folate and 30 mg/day of iron in the second and third trimester to ensure maternal and fetal health. Blood glucose levels, ketone production, appetite, and weight gain are used to adjust the meal plan throughout the pregnancy.

Exercise

Pregnancy is not a time to introduce strenuous exercise. The guidelines of the American College of Obstetricians and Gynecologists are usually the recommendations followed *(Table 6-4)*. Regular, moderate level exercise is beneficial to both mother and baby.

Insulin

Many regimens of insulin administration are used to achieve the blood glucose goals. The most important consideration is to keep activity and the timing and content of meals consistent so that insulin doses can be adjusted to keep up with the changing requirements that occur during pregnancy. Early in the pregnancy, twice daily injections of intermediate- and rapid-acting insulins are often adequate to control blood glucose levels. The early weeks of pregnancy are usually associated with a decrease in insulin requirements from the

---

TABLE 6-4
Exercise During Pregnancy in Women with Diabetes

Maternal heart rate should not exceed 140 beats per minute.

Strenuous activities should not exceed 15 minutes in duration.

No exercise should be done supine after the fourth month of gestation.

Exercises that incorporate the Valsalva maneuver should be avoided.

Caloric intake should be adequate to meet the extra energy needs of pregnancy and the exercise performed.

Maternal core temperature should not exceed 38°C.

Source: Reprinted with permission from Lebovitz, H. (Ed.). (1991). *Therapy for Diabetes Mellitus and related disorders* (p. 19). Copyright © 1991 by the American Diabetes Association, Inc.

---

amount required before conception. Therefore, pregnant women should be especially alert to signs and symptoms of hypoglycemia. They may need to decrease their doses of insulin.

After 24–28 weeks, counterregulatory hormones cause a dramatic increase in the amount of insulin required. At this time, often once- or twice-daily doses of intermediate- or long-acting insulin are combined with doses of rapid-acting insulin before meals to allow for the needed adjustments. By the third trimester, dosages two to three times those required before pregnancy are often needed. An insulin infusion pump is an efficient way to achieve normal or near-normal blood glucose levels.

Monitoring During Pregnancy, Labor, and Delivery

In the first trimester and in the early part of the second trimester, sonography of the fetus provides confirmation of gestational age and helps detect certain malformations. Throughout the pregnancy, sonography is used to assess the growth of the fetus and the volume of amniotic fluid.

At about 16–17 weeks of pregnancy, a blood test to determine the concentration of serum a-feto-protein is done to detect any fetus at risk for a neural tube defect. If the concentration is abnormally high, further testing is done.

In the third trimester, fetal activity is monitored by the mother. One method is to count fetal movements for a specified period.

A nonstress test is done to help determine whether the fetus is doing well in utero and to assess for risk of fetal demise. A biophysical profile, which consists of five components, is another test used to evaluate the adaptation of the fetus and risks. When the nonstress test shows no reaction, a contraction stress test is done to assess how the fetal heart rate responds to mild uterine contractions.

An amniocentesis may be done to assess fetal lung maturity. The goal is to allow the pregnancy to progress to term as long as fetal health does not appear to be compromised and no maternal complications such as preeclampsia occur. Diabetes in pregnancy is not considered an independent factor for either cesarean section or the induction of labor.

The goals of managing diabetes during labor are to provide adequate carbohydrate intake to meet the mother's energy requirements and maintain maternal blood concentration in the range of 70–100 mg/dl while preventing ketosis. Usually a solution of glucose is infused continuously, and blood glucose levels are monitored frequently. Insulin is also given, either by subcutaneous injection or an intravenous infusion. These measures also prevent undue increases in fetal insulin secretion before delivery and decrease the risk of neonatal hypoglycemia.

Postpartum Management

An immediate decrease in the insulin requirements occurs in the postpartum period. This change in requirements lasts a variable amount of time until prepregnancy requirements are reestablished. If insulin requirements remain high, the mother may have an underlying infection. If the mother is breast-feeding, the nutritional requirements are the same as those recommended for the third trimester of pregnancy.

Both an increased risk of embolism and an increase in the concentration of blood glucose may occur with the use of oral contraceptives containing estrogen and progesterone. These factors must be carefully evaluated by women with diabetes and their physicians when family planning and contraception are being considered.

GESTATIONAL DIABETES

Gestational Diabetes Mellitus is defined as carbohydrate intolerance of variable severity with onset or first recognition during the current pregnancy (Coustan, 1991). Previously all pregnant women were screened for gestational diabetes. Currently women at low risk (e.g., under 25, normal body weight, no family history of diabetes, do not belong to an ethnic/racial subgroup with high incidence of diabetes) are not screened. The ADA (1999) recommends that all pregnant women over the age of 25 be screened for gestational diabetes at 24–28 weeks of gestation. Any woman who has a history suggestive of previous or current glucose intolerance is screened at the first prenatal visit.

The initial screening involves a 50-gram 1-hour oral glucose challenge administered without regard to time of day or interval since the woman's last meal. If the concentration of blood glucose is equal to or greater than 140 mg/dl, a 100-gram 3-hour oral glucose tolerance test is done. The woman should fast the night before the test (8–14 hours) after 3 days of unrestricted diet and activity. A diagnosis of gestational diabetes is made if two or more of the venous plasma glucose levels meet or exceed the values given in *Table 6-5*. Women with a clinical history of glucose intolerance but normal results in the screening test are screened again in the 32nd–34th week of pregnancy.

Gestational diabetes has implications for both mother and fetus. In one study, perinatal mortality was 6.4% in pregnancies in women with untreated gestational diabetes and 1.5% in pregnancies in nondiabetic women. Rates of risk can be reduced to those of the general population when proper management is instituted (Coustan, 1991). Women with gestational diabetes have an increased risk for perinatal loss when this condition goes untreated. The disorder is also associated with macrosomatia, hypoglycemia, hypocalcemia, polycythemia vera, and hyperbilirubinemia. The maternal implication of gestational diabetes is a high risk for diabetes after pregnancy.

Treatment

Treatment consists of ensuring normal blood glucose control through diet and use of insulin (if needed). The goals and strategies for dietary management are the same as those outlined for diabetes in pregnancy. Because many women who have gestational diabetes are overweight at the time it is diagnosed, particular attention is paid to caloric intake. However, weight loss is not advised. After pregnancy, counseling is aimed at attaining and maintaining desirable body weight.

Insulin therapy may be needed to ensure normalization of blood glucose levels and to prevent macrosomatia in the newborn. Insulin therapy is usually begun if the fasting blood glucose levels exceed 105 mg/dl or the 2-hour postprandial levels

---

TABLE 6-5

Criteria for Diagnosis of Gestational Diabetes

After an oral glucose load of 100 grams, the diagnosis of gestational diabetes may be made if two plasma glucose values equal or exceed the following:

Time After Glucose Load (hour)	Glucose Value (mg/dl)
0 (fasting; baseline)	105
1	190
2	165
3	145

Source: Rifkin, H. (Ed.). (1985). *The physician's guide to type II diabetes (NIDDM): Diagnosis and treatment* (p. 10). Copyright © 1985 by the American Diabetes Association, Inc.

---

are more than 120 mg/dl. When insulin is prescribed, only human insulins should be used.

Fetal monitoring tests as outlined earlier are used for women with gestational diabetes. Spontaneous labor at term is the goal unless fetal or maternal health is endangered. The goals of management during labor are the same as for women who had diabetes before they became pregnant. Normal blood glucose levels are often maintained during labor without the need for insulin. Insulin treatment is discontinued in the postpartum period. Women who continue to have increases in the concentration of blood glucose after the birth of the baby can be managed with diet, oral hypoglycemic agents, or insulin as needed.

The risk of subsequent diabetes for women who have gestational diabetes is high, and testing for glucose intolerance at a postpartum visit is recommended (Coustan, 1991). All women who have had gestational diabetes should be counseled on the importance of attaining and maintaining ideal body weight, having annual blood glucose tests, and contacting their health provider if signs and symptoms of high blood glucose levels occur.

EXAM QUESTIONS

CHAPTER 6
Questions 46–55

46. A barrier related to normal aging that might prevent an elderly person with diabetes from engaging in self-care behaviors is most apt to be a decrease in

    a. interest.

    b. visual acuity.

    c. problem-solving skills.

    d. ability to learn new behaviors.

47. If a person with insulin-treated diabetes plans to travel and meal times will be unpredictable, management instructions might include which of the following?

    a. Decrease usual insulin dose by 50%.

    b. Carry all meals along.

    c. On travel days, eat only protein and complex carbohydrates.

    d. Change from longer acting insulin to sliding-scale regular insulin.

48. During preconception counseling, a female with diabetes would be told which of the following?

    a. The baby has a sixfold risk for type 1 diabetes.

    b. Even with good blood glucose control, the risk of spontaneous abortion is twice that of women without diabetes.

    c. Retinopathy, even though treated, is a contraindication to pregnancy.

    d. Good glycemic control early in the pregnancy may decrease the risk of congenital anomalies.

49. When should pregnant women with diabetes monitor their urine for the presence of ketones?

    a. At the first voiding in the morning and anytime the blood glucose level is more than 150 mg/dl.

    b. Before and after each meal.

    c. Whenever the blood glucose level is checked.

    d. At the last voiding before bedtime and anytime the blood glucose level is more than 150 mg/dl.

50. Which of the following are considered the most important predictors of adverse outcomes associated with diabetes and pregnancy?

    a. The patient's age at the time diabetes is diagnosed, number of pregnancies, metabolic control.

    b. The patient's age at conception, duration of diabetes, presence of vascular disease.

    c. The patient's age at conception, number of pregnancies, presence of neuropathy.

    d. Poor metabolic control, self-neglect, presence of vascular disease.

51. What is the definition of gestational diabetes?

    a. Carbohydrate intolerance with onset or first recognition during pregnancy.

    b. Pregnancy in a woman with preexisting diabetes.

    c. Development of diabetes in the fetus during gestation.

    d. Presence of carbohydrate intolerance in newborn.

52. During growth spurts, children with diabetes may require which of the following?

    a. Fewer calories and more insulin.

    b. More calories and more insulin.

    c. Fewer calories and less insulin.

    d. More calories and less insulin.

53. A pregnant woman with diabetes is more likely to have a normal birth if near-normal blood glucose levels are maintained at which time during the pregnancy?

    a. Throughout the pregnancy.

    b. Before conception and throughout pregnancy.

    c. Before conception and throughout the first trimester.

    d. Throughout the first trimester.

54. Congenital malformations in infants of mothers with diabetes occur during which gestational period?

    a. Second trimester

    b. Last 7 weeks

    c. First trimester

    d. Third trimester

55. The risk of postoperative myocardial infarction in the diabetic patient compared to the patient without diabetes is

    a. the same for both groups.

    b. lower in the diabetic patient.

    c. higher in the non-diabetic patient.

    d. higher in the diabetic patient.

CHAPTER 7

ACUTE COMPLICATIONS OF DIABETES

CHAPTER OBJECTIVE

After completing this chapter, the reader will be able to discuss the signs, symptoms, and treatment of acute complications of diabetes, including loss of blood glucose control, including hypoglycemia, illness, hyperglycemia, diabetic ketoacidosis (DKA), hyperglycemic hyperosmolar nonketotic syndrome (HNKS), and infections.

LEARNING OBJECTIVES

After studying this chapter, the reader will be able to:

1. Specify the signs and symptoms of three levels of hypoglycemia.

2. Recognize common causes of hypoglycemia.

3. Indicate appropriate interventions for patients with hypoglycemia.

4. Specify medications that cause hyperglycemia.

5. Recognize the guidelines for patients for diabetes management during illness and on sick days.

6. Recognize appropriate treatment for patients with diabetes who have experienced the dawn phenomenon.

7. Recognize appropriate treatment for severe DKA.

8. Recognize the signs and symptoms of HNKS.

9. Specify precipitating factors for DKA and HNKS.

10. Indicate treatment of HNKS.

INTRODUCTION

The acute complications of diabetes discussed in this chapter require immediate attention and can be life threatening. Hypoglycemia is the most common and life threatening complication, and prompt recognition and treatment are essential. Hyperglycemia stemming from uncontrolled blood glucose levels can lead to two metabolic crises, DKA and HNKS. Although the morbidity and mortality caused by these acute complications are declining, DKA and HNKS still present a serious and significant problem. Intervention should focus on early recognition and prompt treatment of the prodromal conditions, such as loss of blood glucose control and infections, that may lead to these crises.

HYPOGLYCEMIA

Hypoglycemia, insulin reaction, and insulin shock are all terms denoting too little glucose in the bloodstream. In patients with diabetes managed by diet alone, hypoglycemia is rare. It can and does occur in patients taking oral hypoglycemic agents. However, hypoglycemia is the most common acute complication of therapy in patients who take insulin.

The incidence of hypoglycemia varies according to the intensity of treatment and the patient's knowledge. The statistics quoted by some authorities are shocking. According to Pickup and Williams (1991), hypoglycemic coma occurs at least once in more than 30% of patients who use insulin and eventually results in death in 3–4%. The severity of hypoglycemic reactions is variable, and the patients with type 1 diabetes often experience many milder hypoglycemic episodes. The typical patient with type 1 diabetes who uses two daily injections of insulin most likely will experience approximately one episode of hypoglycemia per week or about 1,482 episodes over 30 years (Santiago et al., 1991). All patients must learn the signs and symptoms of hypoglycemia, the risks involved, and measures of prevention and treatment.

Definitions of Hypoglycemia

Hypoglycemia is usually defined biochemically as a whole blood glucose level less than 50 mg/dl with or without the presence of other signs or symptoms. However, many episodes of hypoglycemia are sensed at blood glucose levels above this value, and others go undetected, especially during the night, for lower levels. Therefore, this clinical definition, although precise, is not the most useful. For example, some patients remain alert and fully functional at blood glucose levels of 40 mg/dl, whereas in others, coma develops at this level. Clinical definitions of hypoglycemia are usually used as the more practical method of defining the severity of hypoglycemia.

Mild Hypoglycemia

Mild hypoglycemia is defined as an episode in which the patient feels sensations related to: (1) activation of the adrenergic system, such as tachycardia, palpitations, or shakiness; (2) or to activation of the cholinergic system, such as a cold sweat or pallor; or (3) experiences the effects of hypoglycemia on the nervous system, such as an inability to concentrate, dizziness, headache, hunger, or blurred vision. Adrenergic signs and symptoms of hypoglycemia can sometimes be elicited by a rapid decrease in the concentration of blood glucose even in the absence of biochemical hypoglycemia, for example, a decrease in blood glucose from 200 to 100 mg/dl (11 to 5.5 mmol/L) over 1 hour (White, Gingerich, Levandoski, Cryer & Santiago, 1985).

Cognitive deficits usually do not accompany mild reactions, and the impairment is not severe enough to interfere with patients' normal activities. Patients are capable of self-treatment, and a decrease in these mild signs and symptoms occurs within 10–15 minutes after the ingestion of 10–15 grams of simple carbohydrate.

Moderate Hypoglycemia

Moderate hypoglycemia is defined as an episode of hypoglycemia that is associated with: (1) neuroglycopenia or impaired function of the central nervous system due to cellular deprivation of glucose; and (2) adrenergic signs and symptoms. Common symptoms include mood changes, irritability, decreased attentiveness, drowsiness, somnolence, confusion, slurred speech, inappropriate behavior, and impairment of motor function.

Patients are usually alert enough to seek self-treatment but because of the symptoms may require assistance in treatment. Moderate hypoglycemic reactions produce longer lasting and somewhat more severe signs and symptoms than mild hypoglycemic reactions and often require a second dose of simple carbohydrate.

Severe Hypoglycemia

Severe hypoglycemia is defined as an episode of hypoglycemia in which the patient's impairment of neurologic function is severe enough to require the assistance of another person for treatment. Severe reactions are characterized by unresponsiveness, loss of consciousness, coma, and seizures. Oral carbohydrates may be used, but often glucagon or intravenous glucose is needed for treatment.

Physiologic Responses to Hypoglycemia

In acute hypoglycemia induced by insulin, spontaneous recovery occurs if the secretion of glucose counterregulatory hormones, primarily glucagon and epinephrine, are sufficient to cause an increase in the level of glucose in the bloodstream (Cryer, White & Santiago, 1986). If the period of hypoglycemia is prolonged, growth hormones and cortisol also contribute to the recovery. However, insulin levels are the most important factor in recovery from hypoglycemia. High levels blunt the body's recovery efforts, and lower levels enhance the recovery.

When hypoglycemia occurs, secretion of glucagon stimulates the release of stored glycogen as glucose from the liver. This release increases the concentration of glucose in the blood. Secretion of glucagon often becomes impaired after 2–5 years in patients with type 1 diabetes.

The role of epinephrine in recovery from hypoglycemia is secondary when glucagon secretion is adequate. Epinephrine is the primary means of recovery when glucagon secretion is inadequate. Epinephrine enhances recovery from hypoglycemia by two mechanisms. It increases hepatic production of glucose and decreases utilization of the sugar. Diminished secretion of epinephrine, which is probably the result of autonomic (sympathetic) neuropathy, usually occurs later than glucagon deficiency in the course of diabetes.

If both glucagon and epinephrine secretory responses to hypoglycemia are deficient, a condition known as defective counterregulation (Cryer et al., 1986) occurs. In this situation, the normal rescue mechanisms of the body no longer function. Patients with this condition are at risk for severe, recurrent hypoglycemia. Defective counterregulation is thus a limiting factor in tight control of diabetes, because the risks of serious episodes of hypoglycemia are usually considered to outweigh the benefits of improved blood glucose levels.

Potential Effects of Hypoglycemia

Mild hypoglycemia is usually only a mild nuisance. However, it can cause overeating if it becomes a regular occurrence, and it can contribute to erratic blood glucose control, hyperglycemia, and weight gain.

Moderate or severe hypoglycemia can be disabling in several ways. Hypoglycemia that interferes with cognitive functioning can become serious. Work or school performance can be affected, and physical dangers include the possibility of accidents while the patient is driving or using machinery. With repeated or prolonged episodes of moderate or severe hypoglycemia, irreparable damage to the central nervous system can occur. Such damage is particularly a concern in young children. Their central nervous system is not yet mature, and the deprivation of glucose is especially harmful. Interpersonal relationships can also be severely affected, as when episodes of hypoglycemia cause embarrassment or fear.

Some patients acquire a phobic fear of hypoglycemia that can lead to overeating or to undertreatment with insulin. If a patient insists on maintaining high concentrations of blood glucose to avoid hypoglycemia, the risks for ketoacidosis and long-term complications are greatly increased. Some patients adopt a nonchalant attitude with an inappropriate lack of concern about hypoglycemia that can put them at great risk for severe recurrent hypoglycemia.

Causes of Hypoglycemia

The causes of hypoglycemia can often be determined by examining the events of the hours preceding the event *(Table 7-1)*.

TABLE 7-1
Common Causes of Hypoglycemia

Insulin errors (inadvertent or deliberate)

Reversal of morning and evening doses

Reversal of short- and intermediate-acting insulin

Improper timing of insulin in relation to food

Excessive insulin dosage

Erratic or altered absorption of insulin

More rapid absorption from exercising limbs

Unpredictable absorption from hypertrophied injection sites

Use of more purified insulin preparations or change from mixed-species to single-species or human insulin

Diet

Omitted or inadequate amount of food

Timing errors: late snacks or meals

Exercise

Unplanned activity

Prolonged duration or increased intensity of activity

Alcohol and drugs

Impaired hepatic gluconeogenesis associated with alcohol intake

Impaired mentation associated with alcohol, marijuana, or cocaine

Source: Reprinted with permission from Sperling, M. (Ed.). (1988). *The physician's guide to insulin-dependent (type I) diabetes: Diagnosis and treatment* (p. 72). Copyright © 1988 by the American Diabetes Association, Inc.

Insulin Errors and Alterations in Insulin Absorption

Injection of insulin without: (1) adequate carbohydrate intake or (2) normal glucose counterregulatory mechanisms is the most common cause of hypoglycemia. Too much insulin can be predicted to occur at certain times of the day, depending on the peak action times of the insulin. Too much insulin is also possible when attempts are being made to maintain the concentration of blood glucose at near-normal levels. Other potential causes can be a change in insulin type, errors in administration, and altered absorption rates. Longer acting insulins such as Ultralente and oral hypoglycemic agents can cause hypoglycemia. Prolonged hypoglycemia is common in elderly patients who use chlorpropamide (Diabenese).

Dietary Factors

Inadequate or poorly timed absorption of food can also cause hypoglycemia. Delayed or skipped meals or meals with inadequate carbohydrate content can be reasons for low levels of blood glucose. Gastrointestinal neuropathy (gastroparesis), manifested by delays in gastric emptying time, and impaired absorption are also causative factors.

Exercise

Exercise (see chapter 3) has both an immediate and a prolonged effect on lowering blood glucose levels. The immediate effect of exercise is to accelerate the absorption of insulin from subcutaneous tissue because of increased blood flow. The increase in insulin in the bloodstream inhibits the release of glucose from the liver that normally occurs in response to exercise. This immediate effect predisposes exercisers to hypoglycemia during and shortly after exercise if adequate snacks are not consumed. Prolonged strenuous exercise depletes glycogen stores and can result in lower blood glucose levels for as long as 12–24 hours. The institution of a physical conditioning program that increases insulin sensitivity and reduces insulin requirements can also cause hypoglycemia.

Alcohol

Drinking alcohol, especially if food is not eaten, leads to hypoglycemia because of the inhibiting effect of alcohol on the release of glucose from the liver. This effect can occur with as little as 2–3 ounces (60–90 ml) of alcohol.

Hormonal Changes

In women, the hormonal changes associated with the onset of menstruation, the first trimester of pregnancy, and the immediate postpartum period are physiologic causes of an increase in risk for hypoglycemia. During these times, women must be alert for changes in the need for insulin to prevent overinsulinization.

Autonomic Neuropathy

Autonomic neuropathy that causes a decrease in the release of epinephrine in response to hypoglycemia may contribute to an increase in the severity of the episode. In addition, patients may eventually have "hypoglycemia unawareness" if the initial warning signs and symptoms of mild hypoglycemia no longer occur. This phenomenon also seems to occur in patients who maintain their concentration of blood glucose in the normal ranges and become more tolerant of a lower blood glucose level.

Medications

Certain medications *(Table 7-2)* that may be used for treatment of concurrent medical problems may also promote or contribute to hypoglycemia. Drugs such as propranolol (Inderal®) may mask the early warning signs and symptoms associated with hypoglycemia and place patients at risk for more severe hypoglycemia.

Treatment of Hypoglycemia

Treatment of hypoglycemia depends on the severity of the complication.

Mild Hypoglycemia

Treatment for mild hypoglycemia is ingestion of 10–15 grams of simple oral carbohydrate. Four to six ounces (120–180 ml) of carbohydrate-containing liquid (e.g., fruit juice), 6–10 Lifesavers, and a tablespoon (15 ml) of honey or Karo syrup all contain sufficient short-acting carbohydrate to treat a mild reaction. If the episode occurs during the night, the initial treatment should be followed by ingestion of a longer acting mixture of carbohydrate, protein, and fat (8 oz of milk [240 ml] or 4 oz of milk and a few crackers) to sustain the increase in the concentration of blood glucose and prevent further hypoglycemia during the rest of the night.

Some health professionals advocate treatment with simply a small amount of food (e.g., milk). Commercially available glucose tablets are useful, because they are premeasured and prepackaged and help prevent overtreatment. Glucose gel products or small tubes of cake frosting are also convenient and easily carried. Chocolate and ice cream should be discouraged as a treatment, because the fat content could retard the absorption of sugar and they can contribute to weight gain.

Because of the risk that mild hypoglycemia could progress to a more severe reaction, all episodes should be treated immediately. If patients are driving a car or participating in an activity in which hypoglycemia could present a hazard, they

---

TABLE 7-2

Drugs That Cause Hypoglycemia

Alcohol
Alcohol-induced hypoglycemia usually is the result of decreased hepatic glucose output, which ordinarily protects against fasting and postprandial hypoglycemia.

Bishydroxycoumarin
This drug may prolong the metabolic activity of sulfonylurea agents. When anticoagulation is needed in a patient being treated with a sulfonylurea, warfarin should be used.

Phenyibutazone and other pyrazalone derivatives (sulfinpyrazone, oxyphenbutazone)
These agents may potentiate the action of sulfonylureas by displacing sulfonylurea from plasma protein binding sites, by prolonging sulfonylurea half-life, or by decreasing urinary excretion of sulfonylurea compounds or their metabolites.

Salicylates
Large doses of aspirin (4 grams or more per day) may have a primary hypoglycemic effect. They may also displace sulfonylurea drugs from their binding sites and enhance hypoglycemic activity.

Sulfonamides
The sulfonamides probably prolong the metabolic activity of sulfonylurea agents by displacing them from protein-binding sites. Alternative antibacterial agents should be used in patients taking sulfonylurea drugs.

Beta-adrenergic blockers
Nonselective: **Propranolol, Nadolol, Timolol, Pindolol**
Cardioselective: **Metoprolol, Atenolol**
The beta-adrenergic blocking agents prevent rapid hepatic glycogenolytic responses, which normally correct insulin-induced or spontaneous hypoglycemia.

Monoamine oxidase inhibitors
These agents probably prolong sulfonylurea half-life via competition for enzymes.

Source: Reprinted with permission from Rifkin, H. (Ed.). (1985). *The physician's guide to type II diabetes (NIDDM): Diagnosis and treatment* (p. 81). Copyright © 1985 by the American Diabetes Association, Inc.

---

should stop, treat the hypoglycemia, and wait 10–15 minutes for full recovery before resuming the driving or the other activity.

Moderate Hypoglycemia

Patients with moderate hypoglycemia often respond to the oral carbohydrates listed previously but may require more than one treatment and may take longer to recover. Patients are advised to wait 10–15 minutes after taking the carbohydrate and then eat some additional food (e.g., low-fat milk, cheese, and crackers), after the initial signs and symptoms resolve. After treatment, they should wait 10–30 minutes before resuming activity.

Measuring blood glucose levels during and after the initial treatment help in evaluating the effectiveness of treatment. Even after the increase in the concentration of blood glucose to values greater than 100 mg/dl, posthypoglycemic signs of

symptoms of shakiness, fatigue, slurred speech, agitated behavior, or transitory hemiparesis may persist for an hour or longer.

Severe Hypoglycemia

Severe hypoglycemia with impaired consciousness or an inability to swallow is best treated by the administration of glucagon (1mg for adults and children more than 5 years old, 0.5 mg for children less than 5 years old) or 50% glucose intravenously. If these are not available, glucose gel products, honey, syrup, or jelly can be placed between the patient's cheek and gum. Once the patient responds to intravenous glucose or glucagon, it is advisable to administer some simple sugar until nausea (if present) subsides, and then the patient should eat a small meal or snack.

It is important to monitor blood glucose levels frequently for several hours after an episode of severe hypoglycemia to ensure against recurrent hypoglycemia and prevent overtreatment. After a severe episode, patients should notify and consult a health team member to determine the cause and corrective actions needed.

Measures to Help Prevent Hypoglycemia

Teaching patients and their families about the signs and symptoms, causes, and prompt treatment of hypoglycemia is the most important factor in preventing serious and recurrent episodes of hypoglycemia. It must be understood that delays in meals and snacks or eating less than planned puts patients at risk for hypoglycemia. For this reason, patients with diabetes should always carry a fast-acting source of carbohydrate. All patients with diabetes should carry an identification card with information about their treatment or wear a Medic-Alert bracelet or necklace. Family members should be instructed how to use glucagon and how to monitor blood glucose levels. Patients should measure blood glucose levels or treat themselves for hypoglycemia if any signs or symptoms of the complication occur. Hypoglycemia detected by monitoring blood glucose levels, even when no signs or symptoms are present, should also be treated.

Hypoglycemia that occurs on a regular basis requires some adjustment to the treatment plan. Periods of exercise should be timed properly (see chapter 3), and replacement of carbohydrate must be adequate (see chapter 2) to prevent hypoglycemia. Blood glucose levels should be monitored before, during, and after strenuous or irregular exercise. Periodic monitoring of the nocturnal (3 a.m.) concentration of blood glucose is helpful in preventing hypoglycemia when the patient makes adjustments in the evening dose of insulin, if strenuous physical activity has occurred, and during periods of erratic activity or food intake.

Patients should also know that their signs and symptoms of hypoglycemia may change over time

and may result in hypoglycemia unawareness. If hypoglycemia unawareness develops, blood glucose monitoring should be done more often, and blood glucose goals may need adjustments to prevent hypoglycemia.

HYPERGLYCEMIA

Rebound hyperglycemia (hypoglycemia begets hyperglycemia) that occurs after a hypoglycemic episode is known as the Somogyi phenomenon *(Table 7-3)*. During hypoglycemia, the body secretes the counterregulatory hormones (glucagon, epinephrine, growth hormone, and cortisol). This surge in hormones, together with falling insulin levels and the increase in glucose production from the liver, causes an excessive increase in the concentration of blood glucose. In addition, because of the counterregulatory hormones, insulin resistance may occur for a period of 12–48 hours.

Most often a pattern becomes established in which unrecognized nocturnal hypoglycemia results in elevated fasting levels of blood glucose. In response to these increases, the patient increases the insulin dose, and the problem worsens. A cycle of overinsulinization may result in which more hypoglycemia is followed by ever-increasing hyperglycemia that does not respond to treatment. Often patients have nightmares and night sweats, with elevated fasting levels of blood glucose, and ketones in the urine.

The concentration of blood glucose should be measured between 2 a.m. and 4 a.m. and again at 7 a.m. If the concentration is low (e.g., 20–60 mg/dl) between 2 a.m. and 4 a.m. and more than 180–200 mg/dl at 7 a.m., rebound hyperglycemia is occurring. The most effective treatments usually are to: (1) lower the insulin dosage; (2) take the presupper dose of intermediate-acting insulin at bedtime; and/or (3) change or increase the bedtime snack.

TABLE 7-3
When to Suspect Rebound Hyperglycemia

Unstable glucose readings characterized by daily fluctuations between hypoglycemia and severe
hyperglycemia

Increasing glucose levels despite increasing insulin doses

Awakening with ketonuria in the absence of glycosuria

Awakening with headaches, restless sleep, nightmares, or enuresis (all suggestive of nocturnal hypoglycemia); nausea or vomiting without explanation

High insulin doses

Children: more than 1.0 unit $\cdot$ kg^{-1} $\cdot$ day^{-1} *

Adolescents: more than 1.5 units $\cdot$ kg^{-1} $\cdot$ day^{-1}

Adults: more than 1.5 units $\cdot$ kg^{-1} $\cdot$ day^{-1}

*Alternative notations: units/(kg $\cdot$ day) and units/kg/day.

Source: Reprinted with permission from Sperling, M. (Ed.). (1988). *The physician's guide to insulin-dependent (type I) diabetes: Diagnosis and treatment* (p. 74). Copyright © 1988 by the American Diabetes Association, Inc.

Patterned Hyperglycemia

The key to diabetes management is the achievement of smooth overall control of blood glucose levels, with consistent readings throughout the day and from day to day. Detecting and assessing patterns in blood glucose values can be used as a systematic method of achieving this consistency. A pattern of hyperglycemia becomes apparent when blood glucose levels, measured at the same time each day, show a consistent increase or are consistently low.

In many cases of patterned hyperglycemia, the problem can be solved by using the blood glucose readings to determine possible causes of the hyperglycemia and then making appropriate adjustments in treatment. For example, if the concentration of blood glucose is consistently high when the glucose level is checked at noon, then the events of the morning should be examined to find the cause of the high concentrations. Factors that could contribute to these elevations include the breakfast meal, the morning snack, the rapid-acting insulin

taken before breakfast, and the physical activity of the morning.

In order to assess the situation, each factor should be considered independently. The composition of the breakfast meal (e.g., carbohydrate, protein, and caloric content) may need some adjustment. In this case, a reduction in the size of the breakfast may be needed. Another possible adjustment would be to increase the activity level. The patient could avoid changing the composition or size of the breakfast, because the increased activity would help in using the carbohydrates consumed at breakfast. If a snack is being consumed in the morning, this practice could be discontinued or changed also.

If all these elements, meal, activity, and snack, are well balanced, the final area of adjustment is the dosage of insulin. An increase in the dose of rapid-acting insulin in the morning injection will have an effect on the blood glucose level measured before the noon meal. Small amounts of insulin, in the range of 1–2 units, are generally tried to gradually titrate the blood glucose levels.

If patients and their health care providers use the tools of management, especially blood glucose monitoring, effective interventions can be made to prevent loss of blood glucose control. Achieving consistency in blood glucose readings promotes a feeling of well-being and a sense of confidence.

Some of the medications used in the treatment of other illnesses or conditions may also affect blood glucose levels and cause hyperglycemia *(Table 7-4)*.

The Dawn Phenomenon

One example of patterned hyperglycemia that may occur in patients with diabetes, is called the dawn phenomenon. This phenomenon is an increase in insulin requirements that occurs in many people during the early morning hours. Changes in the level of certain hormones (probably an increase in the secretion of growth hormones and, possibly, cortisol) cause an increase in the concentration of blood glucose, which in turn requires increased levels of insulin to maintain blood glucose at normal levels (Krall & Beaser, 1989).

One way to determine if elevated morning glucose values are due to the dawn phenomenon is to measure the concentration of blood glucose at 3 a.m. and again at 6 a.m. If the reading at 3 a.m. is normal, and the 6 a.m. reading is high, the probable cause is the dawn phenomenon (as discussed earlier, if the 3 a.m. reading is low, and the fasting 6 a.m. reading is high, the probable cause is the Somogyi phenomenon).

The treatment for the dawn phenomenon is to change the timing of the intermediate dose of insulin the evening before. If the patient is taking NPH insulin before dinner, moving the timing of the dose to 10 p.m. will most often change the time of the peak insulin level to coincide with the time of the early morning increase in the amount of glucose in the blood and thus improve the morning fasting level of blood glucose.

SICK DAY MANAGEMENT

Colds, flu, infections, injuries, illnesses, surgery, and stressful periods cause increases in blood glucose levels that require immediate intervention to prevent more serious complications due to loss of blood glucose control. The body responds to illness and stress by increasing the secretion of the counterregulatory hormones (glucagon, epinephrine, and cortisol). These hormones exert a catabolic effect and increase the availability of glucose and alternative sources of energy through lipolysis, glycogenolysis, and ketogenesis.

Both the action of these hormones and insufficient insulin to meet the increased needs during illness result in hyperglycemia. In turn, hyperglycemia contributes to osmotic diuresis, and loss of glucose, fluid, and electrolytes occurs. If the patient is not careful in replacing fluids containing electrolytes, more rapid dehydration will occur. During illness, a lack of activity and regularly performed exercise also contributes to increases in blood glucose levels.

Patients with type 1 diabetes may be unable to secrete sufficient basal insulin, and this lack of insulin along with the secretion of the counterregulatory hormones can result in excessive accumulation of ketones and ketoacidosis. Patients with type 2 diabetes may have some ketone production but usually will not become ketoacidotic. The reason for this finding is not clearly understood. It is thought that these patients can produce sufficient insulin to meet basic metabolic needs and prevent excessive lipolysis and ketone production. Patients with type 2 diabetes, especially those who are elderly or debilitated with poor fluid intake, are at risk for HNKS.

Guidelines for Sick Days

Survival skills needed for basic diabetes management should include a knowledge of guidelines

---

TABLE 7-4
Drugs That Cause Hyperglycemia

Glucocorticosteroids
Hydrocortisone and its derivatives
These drugs increase hepatic glucose output via gluconeogenesis. If the patient requires intensive corticosteroid therapy, insulin is usually required.

Oral contraceptives
Glucose metabolism is impaired by the synthetic estrogen, mestranol, which is used in some oral contraceptives. The diabetogenic mechanism is probably increased peripheral resistance.

Oral diuretic agents
Thiazide, Chlorothiazide, Hydrochlorothiazide, Trichlormethiazide
These agents cause both intracellular and extracellular potassium depletion, which decreases insulin secretion.

Sympathomimetic agents
Epinephrine, Norepinephrine, Amphetamines, Ephedrine, Phenylephrine, Phenylpropanolamine
These agents induce hyperglycemia by stimulating glycogenolysis and inhibiting insulin secretion.

Nicotinic acid
Nicotinic acid may aggravate glucose intolerance or type 2 Diabetes Mellitus by producing hepatocellular dysfunction.

Source: Reprinted with permission from Rifkin, H. (Ed.). (1985). *The physician's guide to type II diabetes (NIDDM): Diagnosis and treatment* (p. 80). Copyright © 1985 by the American Diabetes Association, Inc.

---

that are essential for handling sick days. If a patient's self-care is adequate, the risk that development of more serious complications, which often require hospitalization, is minimized.

Monitoring

An unexplained increase in blood glucose levels is often a prodromal indication of impending illness for patients with diabetes. If an unexplained increase occurs, blood glucose levels should be measured more often than usual to prevent dangerously high levels going unnoticed. During illness, the frequency of blood glucose monitoring is usually increased to every 4 hours until signs and symptoms subside. Urine ketone levels should be checked when blood glucose levels are more than 250 mg/dl or when nausea or vomiting occurs. In addition, the patient should monitor (or be monitored for) food and fluid intake, body temperature, weight loss, signs and symptoms of dehydration (especially important in children) and level of consciousness.

Medications

Nonprescription remedies are often used to treat minor illnesses and may affect the concentration of blood glucose, particularly if they are taken often. The amount of sugars and alcohol indicated on the label may vary, and the information may not always be accurate. Cough drops, syrups, and other cold remedies often have high concentrations of sugar. Alcohol is used in the preparation of elixirs and tinctures. Decongestants often contain epinephrine or other sympathomimetic drugs. The labels on these preparations warn against use of the drugs in patients who have diabetes or hypertension.

The contents of these over-the-counter products tend to change frequently (Campbell, 1988). However, most pharmacists keep an updated list of nonprescription preparations that are sugar- or alcohol-free or both. Patients can be best prepared by keeping a supply of commonly needed (e.g., cold and flu remedies) on hand.

Food and Fluid Intake

The risk of dehydration can be decreased by making a conscious effort to increase fluid intake (see chapter 2). For patients who can tolerate their usual meal plan, an increase in calorie-free fluids is helpful. For patients who are nauseated or vomiting, the use of fluids containing both glucose and electrolytes (regular sodas, dilute fruit juices, ice cream, Gatorade, popsicles) is recommended. Small amounts of fluids, taken frequently are usually best tolerated. Approximately 8–12 ounces (240–360 ml) of fluid per hour is recommended. Signs and symptoms, including thirst, dry mouth, and elevated blood glucose levels, may indicate that an increase in fluids is needed.

The risk for starvation ketosis is lessened when a minimum of 100–150 grams of carbohydrate is consumed each day (Benson, 1985). The general guidelines are to consume approximately 15 grams of carbohydrate every 1–2 hours or 50 grams every 3–4 hours in small meals (see chapter 2 for a complete list of replacements for sick days). If blood glucose levels are elevated (e.g., more than 250 mg/dl), it may not be necessary to consume this much carbohydrate, but the guidelines for fluid consumption must be followed.

Insulin

As mentioned previously, the risks of more serious complications developing are minimized if the patient has sufficient insulin to meet the increased needs during illness. Patients with type 1 diabetes may need to increase their dosage of insulin or use supplemental rapid-acting insulin in response to blood glucose readings. The most serious error made by patients with diabetes or their caregivers is to omit insulin because of the patients' inability to eat. Patients with type 2 diabetes may also need supplemental insulin when they are ill, particularly if oral agents are not tolerated because of nausea or vomiting. A plan for management by insulin during sick days should be made by patients and their health care providers before patients become ill.

Medical Care

Contact with the patient's health care provider or physician is recommended during illness to minimize the risk for more serious complications. This practice is particularly important for children and the elderly. Specific situations that require contacting a physician or health care provider immediately are as follows:

- Signs of dehydration, such as dry mucous membranes, poor skin turgor, lethargy, decreased urine output, and weight loss.

- Signs and symptoms of ketoacidosis, such as labored breathing, fruity breath, abdominal pain, increased vomiting, ketones in the urine with blood glucose levels more than 300mg/dl, and lethargy.

- Vomiting or inability to tolerate food that lasts more than 4–6 hours.

- Persistently high blood glucose levels.

- Illness that lasts more than 1–2 days.

- Diarrhea more than five times or for longer than 24 hours.

- Inability of patient or caregiver to manage the illness.

DIABETIC KETOACIDOSIS

The life-threatening condition known as DKA may develop over a period of weeks or in a few hours if diabetes was not previously controlled. With correct treatment, DKA can be resolved in 12–24 hours. In the past, DKA was associated with an extremely high mortality rate, as high as 50–100%. Even today, this complication is the cause of death in 1–10% of patients (Lebovitz, 1991). These deaths occur either because the patient or the patient's family did not seek medical help in time or because medical staff members lacked knowledge and skills.

DKA occurs primarily in type 1 diabetes. An absolute or relative lack of insulin is the most significant cause of DKA. Illness and infection are the precipitating factors in 25–30% of the cases (Funnell, 1998). In some cases, patients omit taking their insulin: (1) as an act of noncompliance; or (2) mistakenly thinking that insulin should not be taken because of mild flu like signs and symptoms; or (3) presence of gastrointestinal illnesses that prevent oral intake. Superimposed stresses (with the production of high levels of counterregulatory hormones) such as emotional trauma, pancreatitis, steroid therapy, surgery, and pregnancy can also be precipitating causes. When insulin is lacking, a vicious cycle begins *(Figure 7-1).*

Progression of Diabetic Ketoacidosis

With insulin deficiency, the first result is a high concentration of blood glucose with glucose spilling into the urine (glycosuria). The patient then experiences polydipsia (up to 3–4 gallons [11–15 L] of fluid daily) and polyuria with the loss of electrolytes. As sodium and potassium are lost in the urine, muscle weakness, extreme fatigue, and malaise occur. The depletion of potassium can also cause cardiac arrhythmias and cardiac arrest. Semistarvation of the cells brings hunger and increased food intake, but profound weight loss of as much as 20–30 pounds (9–13.5 kg) can occur.

Because of a lack of available glucose for energy, fat is broken down at accelerated rates, resulting in the appearance of ketones (acetoacetic acid, ß-hydroxybutyric acid, and acetone) in the blood and urine. Acidosis begins, and Kussmaul's respirations occur as a compensatory mechanism to rid the body of excess carbon dioxide. The fruity odor of acetone becomes evident on the breath. The patient has tachycardia and hypotension with dry mucous membranes. Orthostatic hypotension can occur because of the decreased intravascular volume. Poor skin turgor and "soft eyeballs" are late signs of profound dehydration in adults. Poor skin turgor occurs earlier in children.

Often patients have abdominal pain, which can be mistaken for acute appendicitis. Tenderness on palpation, diminished bowel sounds, and some muscle guarding are usual signs, especially in children. Patients are often nauseated and vomit, which causes a loss of hydrochloric acid and other electrolytes. Severe dehydration, electrolyte imbalance, and acidosis eventually result in coma.

Diagnosis

The laboratory findings used to confirm the diagnosis of DKA are positive results on a test for serum acetone and a low bicarbonate level. Typical laboratory values include the following:

- Increases occur in the level of blood glucose, usually in the range of 300–800 mg/dl. Depending on the severity and duration of DKA, the concentration can be 200–2,000 mg/dl. The degree of increase in the level of blood glucose is not a good index for gauging the severity of DKA. Glucose levels that are only mildly elevated are common, especially in children, pregnant women, and patients who have been vomiting.

- Serum ketones are usually increased to three or more dilutions.

- The pH is low, usually 6.8–7.3, indicating acidosis.

- Serum bicarbonate is usually less than 15 mEq/L.

- Pco2 is usually low, 10–35 mm Hg, reflecting metabolic acidosis due to hyperventilation.

- Urine is positive for glucose and ketones.

- Serum levels of lipids are increased.

- Hematocrit, hemoglobin, and total protein levels are usually elevated because of dehydration.

- White blood cell count is usually elevated, without a left shift, because of dehydration and

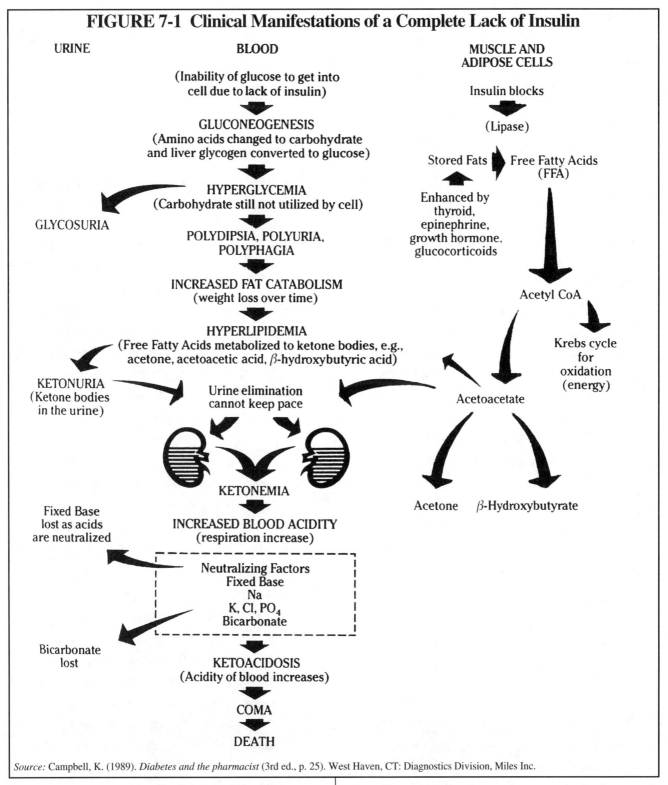

FIGURE 7-1 Clinical Manifestations of a Complete Lack of Insulin

Source: Campbell, K. (1989). *Diabetes and the pharmacist* (3rd ed., p. 25). West Haven, CT: Diagnostics Division, Miles Inc.

stress. A count of more than 20,000 cells or a markedly left shift suggests infection.

- Serum level of sodium is usually low, but it can be normal or high, because the sodium level depends on total body water content.

- Serum level of potassium can be low, normal, or higher than normal. However, a severe total body potassium deficiency almost always occurs.

- Amylase level is usually higher than normal and usually does not indicate pancreatitis, because in patients with DKA, most of the amylase is released by the salivary glands.

- Liver function tests often indicate minor abnormalities. This finding may reflect poor glucose control before the DKA itself occurred. The abnormalities usually resolve when the DKA resolves.

- Serum level of phosphate is usually high initially and then decreases, sometimes to extremely low levels that indicate total body depletion.

- The levels of serum creatinine and blood urea nitrogen may be higher than normal because of dehydration, tissue destruction, or renal disease. When ketones are cleared from the blood, continued elevations in the concentrations of these compounds indicate renal disease.

An electrocardiogram should also be routinely obtained in patients with DKA. The purpose is to provide baseline information, because potassium shifts can be expected. Also myocardial infarctions occur commonly and often silently in patients with diabetes and are often a precipitating factor in DKA.

Treatment

The goals of treatment of DKA are as follows (Davidson, M., 1998):

- Correct fluid and electrolyte disturbances.

- Correct acidosis; for example, normalize bicarbonate levels and pH and clear plasma ketones.

- Provide adequate insulin to establish and maintain normal glucose metabolism.

- Prevent complications of DKA and its treatment.

- Provide for follow-up and education for the patient and the patient's family.

Patients may have various degrees of DKA, from mild to severe, which require different degrees of management.

Mild Cases

Treatment of mild DKA focuses on rehydrating the patient, achieving blood glucose control, and education.

Fluids. Patients may consume oral fluids if the fluids are tolerated, and if vomiting is not occurring. Small amounts of glucose-containing fluids are given at frequent intervals. If the concentration of blood glucose is more than 250 mg/dl, some clinicians prefer to use sugar-free fluids. However, treatment of the dehydration is more important than treatment of the hyperglycemia, and the calories will prevent both ketogenesis and hypoglycemia as blood glucose control is reestablished.

Insulin. Supplemental insulin is required to lower blood glucose levels. Several different approaches are used to calculate insulin dosages. For example, 10–20% of the usual daily dose may be administered as short-acting insulin every 2–4 hours in addition to the usual insulin dose.

Some clinicians prefer to use the intramuscular route, because absorption is more rapid. A dosage of 0.1 unit of regular insulin per kilogram of body weight is administered intramuscularly hourly after blood sugar monitoring until the blood glucose level is less than 250 mg/dl and then subcutaneously every 2–6 hours until blood glucose control is reestablished. Another method is to use a larger dosage of 0.25–0.50 units/kg every 4–6 hours in the same manner.

Follow-up. After the DKA is resolved, follow-up is an essential component of the treatment. Establishing the cause of the complication is helpful in establishing an educational intervention for preventing recurrence of the DKA.

Often, sick day management and stress management are the most helpful in preventing future episodes.

Moderate and Severe Cases

Moderate and severe cases of DKA require immediate emergency treatment. The first step is to ensure an adequate airway and to assess and maintain oxygenation and respiratory function. In most patients, hypovolemia is the most critical problem. Rapid administration of large volumes of fluids is started immediately.

Baseline laboratory data including levels of electrolytes, blood urea nitrogen, creatinine, calcium, phosphorus, serum ketones, and glucose; complete blood cell count; and analysis of arterial blood gases should be obtained immediately. Diagnosis is based on the results of tests for one or a combination of the following: serum ketones, urinary ketones, serum bicarbonate level, arterial pH. An immediate blood glucose level can be obtained by bedside monitoring.

A history should be obtained if possible to collect information important for treatment. Also a physical examination helps ascertain signs and symptoms and other emergency treatment needed. An electrocardiogram, especially lead II, is important to help monitor potassium status and therapy. A nasogastric tube may be inserted in patients who are comatose or have evidence of gastric dilation to prevent aspiration. Catheterization of the urinary bladder generally is used only when the patient's clinical status is so severe that urine output must be monitored.

Fluids. Initial fluid replacement is with ½ NS or NS, depending on the patient's status. The volume depletion is often severe. For adults, initial fluid replacement depends on the degree of dehydration and the cardiovascular status. In general, 1–2 L of fluid is given in the first 1–2 hours, and then the status is reassessed (Davidson, M., 1998).

For children, the amounts are based on kilograms of body weight. The usual amount is 20 ml/kg for 1 hour. If no urination occurs, 20 ml/kg is given in the second and third hour also. The amount used thereafter is calculated by determining the volume needed for maintenance plus deficit.

When the serum glucose level is decreased to 250 mg/dl, the intravenous fluid is changed to a solution of D5/1/2NS or D5/NS. The rate of fluid administration is 150–500 ml/hr, depending on the degree of dehydration and the renal and cardiac status of the patient. Fluid rehydration is usually completed in 12–24 hours (Genuth, 1991).

Potassium. If not treated properly, hypokalemia can result in death. The electrocardiogram (especially lead II) can be helpful in monitoring the level of potassium, because the configuration of the T wave reflects changes in potassium levels as the therapy proceeds *(Figure 7-2)*.

The measured serum level of potassium may

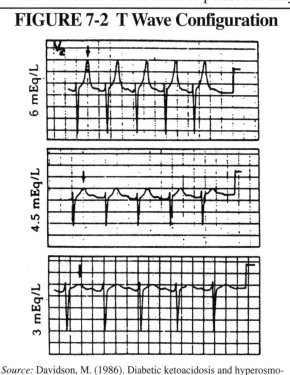

FIGURE 7-2 T Wave Configuration

Source: Davidson, M. (1986). Diabetic ketoacidosis and hyperosmolar nonketotic coma. In *Diabetes Mellitus: Diagnosis and treatment* (2nd ed., p. 225-82). New York: Wiley.

be normal or elevated initially because of the hydrogen ion shift. Hydrogen ions are driven intracellularly during acidosis in exchange for potassium; therefore the serum levels of potassium may be high even though a true intracellular depletion exists. As therapy for DKA begins, potassium values can decline rapidly from the initial readings because of increased glucose utilization associated with administration of insulin, acid-base shifts caused by decreased production of ketoacids, and renal excretion due to improved perfusion of the kidney as a result of rehydration. All patients with urine flow eventually need potassium replacement.

The goal of therapy is to maintain the plasma concentration of potassium at more than 3.5 mEq/L at all times (Genuth, 1991). Both electrocardiographic monitoring and measurements of serum potassium are essential in guiding therapy. Deaths have resulted from hypokalemia and, more rarely, from hyperkalemia (Genuth, 1991). Signs of hypokalemia include skeletal weakness progressing to paralysis, rapid decrease or absence of deep tendon reflexes, shallow gasping respirations (Kussmaul's respirations are deep), and arrhythmias. Potassium chloride is used initially but may be alternated with potassium phosphate later to reduce the chloride load.

Phosphate and magnesium. Plasma levels of phosphate and magnesium are usually normal or elevated at the time of admission for moderate or severe DKA. During treatment, phosphate levels may decrease along with a decrease in the level of magnesium. Clinical consequences of these changes are not significant, and supplementation is generally not indicated unless rhabdomyolysis, deterioration of the central nervous system, cardiac dysfunction, or hemolysis occurs with the initial decrease in the plasma concentration of phosphate. If these changes occur, phosphate supplementation is used (Genuth, 1991).

Sodium bicarbonate. Sodium bicarbonate is often administered when the pH is less than 7.0 or the serum level of bicarbonate is less than 5 mEq/L. However, unless cardiac instability is present or proper fluid and insulin therapy cannot be started, administration of bicarbonate is often not needed and can cause complications of rapid shifts in potassium and pH that can affect the central nervous system (Genuth, 1991). If used, bicarbonate should be given by slow intravenous infusion over several hours. It should be given by bolus injection only in the case of a cardiac arrest (Davidson, M., 1998).

Insulin. All patients with ketoacidosis need insulin. Regular insulin should always be used, because it produces fast results. It takes longer to reverse acidosis than to treat hyperglycemia with insulin.

The most common method of treatment is the insulin drip, a continuous subcutaneous infusion of 0.1–0.2 units of insulin per kilogram of body weight (approximately 2–12 units per hour for adults). A bolus dose of 10 units is recommended to establish a therapeutic level (Genuth, 1991).

An alternative method of treatment is intramuscular (not subcutaneous) injections of low doses of regular insulin. Dosages are calculated in the same way as intravenous infusions.

Glucose levels should decrease approximately 75–100 mg/dl per hour. A more rapid decrease places the patient at risk for cerebral edema. With insulin therapy, glucose concentration falls more rapidly in the blood than in the cerebrospinal fluid. If the concentration of blood glucose decreases too much and too fast, and the brain does not have time to equilibrate, the osmotic gradient pulls water from the blood into the cerebrospinal fluid and brain tissue, resulting in cerebral edema and increased intracranial pressure (Ellenberg & Rifkin, 1983).

As mentioned previously, once the plasma concentration of glucose has reached 250 mg/dl, glucose is added to the replacement fluids. This practice allows continued administration of insulin to resolve the ketosis while protecting the patient from hypoglycemia. When the patient is capable of reliable amounts of oral intake, the insulin infusion is discontinued. Before the infusion is stopped, it is vital to administer 4–10 units of subcutaneous insulin (Genuth, 1991). The half-life of insulin in the bloodstream is approximately 15 minutes, and without subcutaneous insulin, the patient could easily have a recurrence of DKA because of a lack of circulating insulin.

Monitoring and Prevention of Complications

Monitoring blood glucose and potassium levels every 1–2 hours is the key to successful treatment of DKA. The most common treatment errors are: (1) delay in diagnosis; (2) delay in instituting therapy; (3) inadequate fluid replacement; and (4) insufficient or inadequate monitoring.

It is critical for nurses to assess the patient's mental status frequently. If it begins to improve and then deteriorates as the metabolic condition continues to return to normal, cerebral edema should be suspected. If the patient is on a cardiac monitor, indications of hypokalemia include ST segment depression, inverted T waves, and the appearance of U waves following T waves.

After 12–24 hours of treatment, ketones are usually no longer detectable, although in some cases they may be present for several days. Glucose levels generally decrease at a rate of about 100 mg/dl per hour.

Deaths due to DKA occur primarily in older patients and often are due to other medical complications (Gale, Dornan & Tatersall, 1981). The best prognostic indicators are age and depth of coma.

The cause of death is usually infection, arterial thrombosis, or unrelenting shock. The most common complications are aspiration, unrecognized renal tubular necrosis, peripheral or pulmonary edema, cerebral edema, hypokalemia, and unsuccessfully treated precipitating causes (e.g., myocardial infarctions).

Follow-Up and Education

After discharge from the hospital, the patient should be seen in the office of the health care provider within 48 hours and then again in a week, because control is often rather unstable after an episode of DKA, and insulin requirements may change markedly.

The precipitating events and factors that led to the episode of DKA should be reviewed. Education of the patient and the patient's family about patterned hyperglycemia and sick day management should be reinforced. Common errors are not testing for ketones in the urine during illness and omitting doses of insulin when oral intake is decreased. If frequent or repetitive episodes of DKA occur, a referral for psychological intervention is appropriate to ascertain the underlying causes.

HYPERGLYCEMIC HYPER-OSMOLAR NONKETOTIC SYNDROME

A variety of names and acronyms are used for HNKS, including hyperglycemic hyperosmolar nonketotic coma, but a frank coma actually develops in only a few patients. HNKS tends to occur in older patients with type 2 diabetes who are chronically dehydrated or have a chronic low-level concurrent medical illness. Approximately 35% of the cases of HNKS occur in patients in whom diabetes has not been diagnosed (Genuth, 1991). The mortality rate in HNKS is greater than in DKA because of severe metabolic changes, delay in diagnosis, or other medical complications in elderly patients.

The syndrome resembles DKA in extreme volume depletion and hyperglycemia. The hallmark that differentiates DKA from HNKS is the absence of ketosis in patients with the latter. This absence most likely occurs because only small amounts of insulin are needed to prevent ketosis. Ketones may be present in the urine of these patients because of their starvation state, but no acetone will be detected in the plasma. Because no ketosis or acidosis occurs, the gastrointestinal signs and symptoms common in DKA do not occur, and patients do not seek medical care early in the course of the illness.

In HNKS, the osmotic diuresis and dehydration associated with hyperglycemia lead to decreased renal blood flow and allow the concentration of blood glucose to reach extremely high levels. An impaired thirst mechanism or an inability to replace fluids, especially common in the elderly, will exaggerate the tendency for the development of HNKS. Because of the usual course of the illness, patients have a longer time to lose body fluids and thus are more dehydrated than patients with DKA. Concentrations of blood urea nitrogen and serum creatinine are also higher in HNKS than in DKA. The profound dehydration also causes more changes in mentation than is commonly seen in DKA.

Clinical Features and Laboratory Values

Because HNKS is much more insidious than DKA, patients with HNKS typically seek medical care much later and are much sicker than patients with DKA. Their mental status ranges from confusion to complete coma. They may also have generalized or focal seizures, myoclonic jerking, and reversible hemiparesis (Genuth, 1991). Blood pressure is usually low or lower than expected if the patient has a history of hypertension, dehydration is severe, and either hypothermia or hyperthermia may be present.

Typical laboratory values include the following:

- Blood glucose concentration: Above the range of any test strip, usually in the range of more than 800 to 1,000 mg/dl.

- Serum osmolality: more than 350 mOsm/kg.

- Serum sodium concentration: normal or high.

- Blood urea nitrogen and serum creatinine levels: higher than normal.

- Serum potassium concentration: high, normal, or low.

- pH: usually more than 7.3 but may be decreased somewhat.

- Ketones: usually only small amounts present.

Management

The most important aspects of treatment of patients with HNKS are fluid replacement and correction of electrolyte deficits. However, both the type of fluid used and the rate of fluid replacement are matters of controversy. Both hypotonic solutions and isotonic solutions are used, with normal saline solutions being the most commonly utilitzed. As in DKA, fluid replacement depends on the degree of dehydration and the cardiovascular status.

Older patients are more likely to have a compromised cardiovascular status. Therefore, fluid replacement with saline is done cautiously with close monitoring to ensure that the patient will not have congestive heart failure. A patient with history of cardiovascular disease should be monitored with a central venous pressure line or Swan-Ganz catheter. Cerebral edema is a complication of rapid volume replacement. Therefore, the rate of fluid replacement is gradual, about 200–250 ml/hour, and several days are allowed for the patient to fully recover.

Patients with HNKS usually respond to small amounts of insulin. A loading dose of 5–10 units of regular insulin is usually given. This is followed by an insulin drip at a rate of 1–2 units/hour until the

TABLE 7-5

**Comparison of Diabetic Ketoacidosis (DKA) and
Hyperglycemic Hyperosmolar Nonketotic Syndrome (HNKS)**

Characteristic	DKA	HNKS
Onset	Rapid, usually <2 days	Slow usually > one week
Age of Patient	Usually <40 yrs	Usually >40 yrs
Glucose level	Usually <800 mg/dl	Usually >600–1,000 mg/dl
Sodium	Normal or low	Normal or high
Potasssium	High low or normal	High low or normal
Bicarbonate	Low	Normal
Ketones	Large in blood and urine	Small amount to none
Blood pH	Low	Normal
Serum Osmolality	Usually <350 mOsm/kg	Usually >350 mOsm/kg
Prognosis	3–10% mortality	10–20% mortality
Treatment	Insulin in all cases. Fluids	Insulin not required in many cases. Large amounts of fluids.

concentration of blood glucose is stabilized. As is the case in DKA, subcutaneous insulin is started after recovery from HNKS, although patients with HNKS have type 2 diabetes. They may eventually be treated with oral hypoglycemic agents or even diet alone.

Potassium replacement is also necessary in HNKS. The loss of potassium is usually lower than in DKA, because acidosis and vomiting are less. Initial oliguria is common, and potassium is not given until this is resolved. The rate of delivery and the amount of potassium given are generally lower than those used for treatment of DKA. Bicarbonate is not given unless the patient has severe lactic acidosis. Phosphate and magnesium are replaced if indicated.

Because an underlying illness almost always precipitates HNKS, it is crucially important that the illness be determined and treated. Common precipitating causes (Schwartz, 1991) include (1) medications such as steroids, thiazides, dilantin, and ß-blockers; (2) treatments such as peritoneal dialysis and total parenteral nutrition; (3) acute illnesses such as infection, myocardial infarction, and trauma; and (4) chronic illnesses such as cerebrovascular accident, loss of thirst, and psychiatric illnesses.

Follow-Up and Education

After treatment, patients with HNKS should be seen within 2–3 days of discharge and again within 2 weeks to assess whether glucose control is adequate and the precipitating cause has been resolved. With elderly patients, it is important to be sure that a caregiver or spouse is included in the educational process. The importance of sick day management, regular and systematic blood glucose monitoring, and a knowledge of factors related to the development of HNKS cannot be overemphasized.

INFECTIONS

In patients with diabetes, infections often cause deterioration of blood glucose control. They are also a leading cause of metabolic abnormalities leading to DKA and HNKS. Therefore, prompt diagnosis and treatment of infections are absolutely necessary.

Diabetes may predispose patients to certain infections. These include: (1) severe external otitis due to pseudomonas; (2) severe sinus infections due to mucormycosis; (3) urinary tract infections; (4) vulvovaginal candidiasis; (5) tuberculosis; (6) pneumonia due to gram-negative organisms and staphylococci; (7) gallbladder infections; (8) skin and soft-tissue staphylococcal; and (9) necrotizing mixed aerobic and anaerobic infections. For women, candidal infection is often the presenting complaint that leads to a diagnosis of diabetes.

Periodontal and gum infections may also be more common in patients with diabetes than in those without (see chapter 8). The predisposition to infections for patients with diabetes is thought to be related to impairment of leukocyte chemotaxis, phagocytosis, and bactericidal activity as a result of hyperglycemia (Rifkin, 1985).

Treatment and Prevention

Treatment is infection specific. As mentioned previously, it is imperative to determine the cause of the infection and begin treatment immediately. Institution of good blood glucose control is an important factor in improving the body's ability to cope with infection. Compromised circulation, which is prevalent in patients with diabetes, complicates the healing of infections. Prevention involves blood glucose control and hygienic measures and skin care. Pneumococcal and influenza immunizations are often recommended, especially for elderly patients with long-standing diabetes.

EXAM QUESTIONS

CHAPTER 7
Questions 56–65

56. Which of the following is an appropriate response when a patient with diabetes complains of dizziness and hunger and appears pale and unable to concentrate?

    a. Administer 1mg glucagon subcutaneously.

    b. Provide 10–15 g of simple oral carbohydrate.

    c. Provide the next meal immediately.

    d. Administer 50% dextrose intravenously.

57. Which of the following assessments is most important in therapy for severe diabetic ketoacidosis?

    a. Glycosylated hemoglobin level

    b. Potassium level

    c. Amylase level

    d. Phosphate level

58. Which of the following signs and symptoms are characteristic of hypoglycemia?

    a. Deep, rapid breathing

    b. Nausea and vomiting

    c. Cold sweat and pallor

    d. Dehydration

59. Patients with type 1 diabetes should be instructed to contact a physician when vomiting or inability to tolerate food lasts longer than how many hours?

    a. 6

    b. 8

    c. 12

    d. 24

60. Which of the following signs and symptoms are characteristic of hyperglycemic hyperosmolar nonketotic syndrome?

    a. Moderate hyperglycemia, ketosis, dehydration

    b. Kussmaul's breathing, dehydration, ketonuria

    c. Hyperglycemia, ketosis, osmotic diuresis

    d. Severe hyperglycemia, absence of ketosis, dehydration

61. Which of the following steps might a clinician recommend for a patient with diabetes who has experienced the dawn phenomenon?

    a. Measure blood glucose level immediately after exercise.

    b. Take the evening dose of intermediate-acting insulin at 10 p.m.

    c. Decrease the evening dose of intermediate-acting insulin.

    d. Measure blood glucose level at midnight and at 6 a.m.

62. What is the most appropriate goal for a patient with diabetes who has hypoglycemia unawareness?

    a. Discourage vigorous exercise

    b. Maintain tight blood glucose control

    c. Assess for sensory neuropathy

    d. Monitor blood glucose levels frequently

63. Which of the following is a precipitating factor in hyperglycemic hyperosmolar nonketotic syndrome?

    a. Illness

    b. Undiagnosed type 1 diabetes

    c. Increased renal blood flow

    d. Increased lipolysis

64. Prolonged strenuous exercise is a common cause of which complication of diabetes?

    a. Diabetic ketoacidosis

    b. Hyperglycemic hyperosmolar nonketotic syndrome

    c. Hyperglycemia

    d. Hypoglycemia

65. Medications that tend to cause hyperglycemia include which of the following?

    a. Sulfonamides

    b. Propranolol

    c. Salicylates

    d. Epinephrine

CHAPTER 8

LONG-TERM COMPLICATIONS OF DIABETES

CHAPTER OBJECTIVE

After completing this chapter, the reader will be able to discuss the signs, symptoms, and treatments of the long-term complications of diabetes.

LEARNING OBJECTIVES

After studying this chapter, the reader will be able to:

1. Specify ophthalmologic complications associated with diabetes.

2. Indicate recommendations for ophthalmologic examinations for patients with diabetes.

3. Recognize characteristics of various types of diabetic neuropathy.

4. Indicate treatment for various types of diabetic neuropathy.

5. Recognize signs and symptoms of nephropathy associated with type 1 and type 2 diabetes.

6. Indicate treatment for patients with various stages of nephropathy.

7. Specify three macrovascular diseases that affect patients with diabetes.

8. Recognize risk factors for macrovascular diseases in patients with diabetes.

9. Specify important measures that should be taught to patients with diabetes regarding foot care.

10. Indicate the importance of dental care for patients with diabetes.

11. Recognize cutaneous manifestations that occur in patients with diabetes.

INTRODUCTION

Several long-term or chronic complications are associated with diabetes. These include the microvascular diseases of retinopathy, neuropathy, and nephropathy; accelerated macrovascular disease; diabetic foot; cutaneous manifestations; and periodontal disease. These complications account for substantially more morbidity and mortality than the acute complications of diabetes. Fifty percent of hospital admissions for diabetes involve chronic complications (Sinnock, 1985). It has been estimated that diabetes and its associated vascular complications are the fourth leading cause of death in this country (Davidson, 1998). The overall costs for medical and health care, lost wages, and disability due to these complications are several billions of dollars. The impact of these long-term complications on individual patients as well as society at large is tremendous.

Conclusive evidence indicates that good metabolic control helps prevent the development of long-term complications of diabetes (Diabetes Control and Complications Trial [DCCT] Research Group, 1993; UKDPS, 1998). Therefore, it is imperative that every effort be made to help patients achieve and maintain optimal control of blood glucose levels and reduce known risk factors. The long term complications of diabetes fall into two categories; macrovascular disease which is large vessel or atherosclerotic disease and microvascular or small vessel disease.

PATHOPHYSIOLOGY OF COMPLICATIONS

Although the exact relationship between the metabolic abnormalities of diabetes and the morphologic changes that result in long-term complications is not yet clear, several possible mechanisms have been proposed.

Polyol Pathway

Certain tissues in the body are insulin independent (see chapter 1). These tissues (lens, retina, nerves, kidneys, blood vessels, and islets of Langerhans) do not require insulin for glucose to enter the cells. Consequently, glucose enters freely in whatever concentration is present in the bloodstream.

In these tissues, glucose is converted to sorbitol by the enzyme aldose reductase, and sorbitol is converted into fructose by the enzyme sorbitol dehydrogenase. Both sorbitol and fructose are metabolized slowly and diffuse poorly out of the cell. The accumulation of these compounds in the cells causes osmosis. Water is drawn into the cell, resulting in swelling, electrolyte imbalance, and cellular dysfunction.

In peripheral nerves, lower levels of another sugar, myoinositol, alters nerve conduction. Use of a medication that inhibits the enzyme aldose reductase, sorbitol, and diets high in myoinositol results

in some improvement in nerve conduction (Ross, Berstein & Rifkin, 1983).

Basement Cell Membrane Abnormalities

Patients with diabetes have thickening of the capillary basement membranes in the retina of the eye, the glomerulus of the kidney, and the Schwann cells in the nerves. The exact biochemical process by which this occurs is not yet known.

Protein Glycosylation

Hemoglobin and other proteins become glycosylated (glucose is attached to the molecule) in proportion to the concentration of glucose in the bloodstream. This accumulation of glycosylation end products alters the physiologic processes in several ways that contribute to the changes associated with long-term complications.

Atherosclerosis

Atherosclerosis occurs at an earlier age and more often in patients with diabetes than in people without the metabolic disorder. Several reasons account for this difference (Davidson, 1998). Patients with diabetes have an abnormality in the vascular endothelium that allows increased platelet adhesion and aggregation. In addition, the platelets release a substance that causes further thickening and narrowing of the vessel. The high levels of low-density lipoprotein and low levels of high-density lipoprotein commonly found in patients with diabetes result in the formation of plaque at these damaged endothelial sites. Also, the altered coagulation that occurs in some patients with diabetes may promote formation of thrombus.

Blood Glucose Control

The relationship between control of blood glucose levels and the development of long-term complications is no longer a controversial subject. Studies that attempted to ascertain whether good control of blood glucose levels reduced the incidence of complications were marred by several problems. Because of these problems, clinicians and patients were lulled into a false sense of security. They assumed that if complications were destined to develop in a patient with diabetes, complications would develop, despite the level of blood glucose control. The DCCT completed in 1993 conclusively proved that blood glucose control was directly related to the development of microvascular complications in patients with type 1 diabetes (see chapter 10 for further discussion). In this 10-year study, in patients with good control, the risk for diabetic retinopathy was reduced by 76%; the risk for nephropathy (kidney disease), by 50%; and the risk for neuropathy (nerve disease), by 60%. In addition, the risk of cardiovascular disease (macrovascular complications) in these patients was reduced by 35%.

The patients with the reduction in risks achieved an average blood glucose level of 155 mg/dl and an average hemoglobin A1c level of 7.2%. In monitoring patients for the risk of the development of diabetes complications, self-monitoring of blood glucose levels and measurements of glycosylated hemoglobin provide valuable information and a guide for regulating the treatment plan. The DCCT showed that any improvement in blood glucose control has a beneficial effect on reducing the devastating complications of diabetes. In 1998 the results of the UKDPS Study of individuals with type 2 diabetes showed a 35% reduction in microvascular disease and a 25% reduction in death rate in patients who improved blood glucose control.

MICROVASCULAR COMPLICATIONS

The major microvascular complications that occur in diabetes are retinopathy, neuropathy, and nephropathy. The frequent occurrence of these complications together has led to the term triopathy of diabetes. There appears to be a clear relationship between hyperglycemia, the length of time the patient has had diabetes, and the development of microvascular complications.

Diabetic Retinopathy

The development of a problem with sight is probably one of the most well-known and feared complications of diabetes *(Figure 8-1)*. This fear is justified. In the United States, diabetes is the leading cause of new blindness and visual loss in adults. More than 300,000 people are at risk for visual loss from diabetes in the United States alone (ADA Information Services, 1991).

Diabetic retinopathy is the most significant cause of severe visual loss. In addition, other ophthalmologic conditions are associated with diabetes. Some of these complications are related to length of time the patient has had diabetes. Others seem to be related to levels of blood glucose control. All patients with diabetes are vulnerable to these complications whether they have type 1 or type 2 disease.

Over the past several decades, the prevalence of diabetic retinopathy has increased because of the increasing life span of those who have diabetes. Before 1922, retinopathy and blindness due to diabetes were not a problem, because people with diabetes did not have long lives. Diabetic retinopathy is the leading cause of new blindness in Americans between the ages of 20 and 74 years (Davidson, 1998). Legal blindness is defined as visual acuity of 20/200 and may occur as a result of either background (nonproliferative) or proliferative retinopathy.

In patients with type 1 diabetes, retinopathy develops in approximately 50% 7–9 years after diabetes is diagnosed and is present in 90–95% by 15 years after diagnosis (Palmberg et al., 1980). Proliferative retinopathy rarely occurs before 15 years of diabetes, and the highest incidence occurs 15–18 years after the time of diagnosis.

FIGURE 8-1 Basic Structure of the Eye (Profile Views)

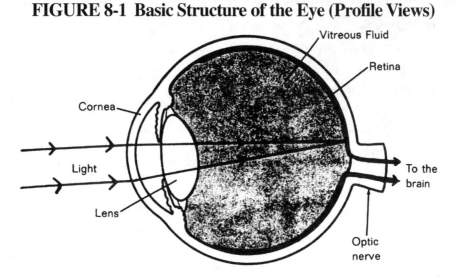

Light passes through the cornea and the lens and is focused on the rear of the eyeball at the layer of the retina. The optic nerve carries the image from the retina to the brain where it is interpreted. The vitreous humor is a clear fluid that keeps the eyeball in constant shape. Four areas of potential trouble are (1) clouding of the lens, which is known as *cataract;* (2) increased pressure of the aqueous, which can damage the optic nerve, a condition known as *glaucoma;* (3) rupture or hemorrhage of the blood vessels in the retina, a condition called *retinitis* or *diabetic retinopathy;* (4) accumulation of fluid in the macula area that has leaked from retinal blood vessels, a condition called *macular edema.*

Source: Krall, L. & Beaser, R. (1989). *Joslin diabetes manual* (p. 271). Philadelphia: Lea & Febiger.

The timing of the onset of retinopathy in patients with type 2 diabetes is less certain. Many have retinopathy at the time of diagnosis, because diabetes often goes undiagnosed in these patients for a long time. In some patients, the diabetes is diagnosed as a result of the discovery of changes in the eye by an ophthalmologist.

Classification

Background retinopathy. In background retinopathy, damage occurs to the microvasculature of the retina of the eye. The exact mechanism of damage is not fully understood. However, it is known that capillaries become damaged, and a dropout of pericytes in the walls of the vessels occurs.

The earliest lesions seen with an ophthalmoscope are microaneurysms, grapelike dilations of capillary-size blood vessels that look like tiny red dots in the retina. Another sign of breakdown in the blood-retina barrier is the appearance of yellowish deposits of lipids that have leaked through the microaneurysms or from the damaged capillaries. These deposits are called hard exudates. Also found are small intraretinal hemorrhages that appear as red smudges on the retina.

Unless macular edema is involved, the patient experiences no symptoms at this stage. This kind of retinopathy is found in almost all patients with diabetes of 25 years' duration or longer. In many cases, it does not progress further (Rifkin, 1985). The most common causes of visual impairment in patients with background retinopathy are macular edema and hard exudates at or near the macula.

Preproliferative retinopathy. Certain retinal lesions represent an advanced form of background retinopathy. When these lesions are found together, the risk for proliferative retinopathy is increased. These lesions include (1) soft exudates or "cotton-wool spots," which are ischemic infarcts in the inner retinal layers; (2) "beading" of the retinal veins, which begin to show tortuosity and bulging over on themselves; and (3) intraretinal microvascular abnormalities, which are dilated capillaries or shunt vessels. These lesions are often found near areas of capillary closure, which can leak and contribute to macular edema. If preproliferative retinopathy is severe, the patient has a 50% chance that proliferative retinopathy will develop within 1 year.

Proliferative retinopathy. Proliferative retinopathy involves the growth of new blood vessels that extend from within the retina onto the inner surface of the retina or into the vitreous humor. These new vessels seem to grow in response to the ischemia present in the damaged retina. They are fragile, so the risk of rupture with hemorrhage is substantial. If bleeding into the preretinal space or vitreous humor occurs, the patient may report "floaters" or "cobwebs" in the field of vision. A sudden loss of vision without warning or pain may be the first evidence of proliferative retinopathy and indicates a major retinal hemorrhage. Growth of fibrous tissue may also accompany the new vascularization and can lead to retinal detachment and permanent loss of vision.

Macular edema. Macular edema is a significant cause of visual loss that may range from mild blurring of vision to 20/200 vision or loss of hand-motion vision. Macular edema involves swelling of the central portion of the retina, the macula. Sometimes, in the advanced stages of retinopathy, fibrous scar tissue extending from the newly formed blood vessels may block the outflow of aqueous humor from the eye, causing a tremendous increase in intraocular pressure ("neovascular glaucoma"), severe pain and loss of vision.

Treatment

Panretinal photocoagulation. Argon-laser photocoagulation is the main method of treating proliferative diabetic retinopathy. In this procedure, multiple laser burns (several hun-

dred) are placed throughout all parts of the retina except the macular area. A 5-year study (Diabetic Retinopathy Study Research Group, 1979) showed that this type of treatment reduced the rate of progression to blindness by 50%. Some loss of vision (from 20/20 to 20/25) occurs in 10% of cases. Patients also have some loss of side vision and increased problems with adaptation to darkness.

The treatment is relatively painless. Most patients require only anesthetic drops. The treatment is done on an outpatient basis, and normal activity can be resumed the next day. Some restrictions in activity, such as no weight lifting, may be necessary.

Focal photocoagulation. Diabetic macular edema is treated with focal argon-laser photocoagulation. This method is similar to "spot-welding" the leaking microaneurysms. In a study by the Early Treatment Diabetic Retinopathy Research Group (1985), focal photocoagulation reduced the rate of visual loss due to macular edema by 50% over a 3-year period.

Vitrectomy. Vitrectomy is a surgical procedure used on eyes with poor vision. General anesthesia is required. The surgeon removes hemorrhage into the vitreous and any fibrous growth and repairs some complex retinal detachments. Vitrectomy is particularly effective in certain cases of advanced proliferative retinopathy. It is usually used only in severely damaged eyes. In about 50–65% of patients who have this procedure, some useful vision is restored.

Medical management. Treatment of hypertension is considered essential for patients with retinopathy, because the eye disease progresses more rapidly in patients with uncontrolled elevation of blood pressure.

Other medical treatments are also being evaluated for retinopathy. These include the use of aspirin (650 mg/day), because it inhibits platelet aggrega-

TABLE 8-1
Guidelines for Eye Care of Patients with Diabetes

Routine care by physician

Examine retinas with direct ophthalmoscope at every visit.

Referral to eye-care specialist

Examine retinas through dilated pupils once a year (this need not be done before puberty).

Referral to ophthalmologist

At the beginning of pregnancy or if planning pregnancy within 12 months

Immediate referral is mandatory (preferably to an ophthalmologist specializing in retinal disease) if any of the following are present.

New vessels on the disk (NVD) greater than ~25% of the optic disk area

Any NVD with preretinal or vitreous hemorrhage

New vessels elsewhere (NVE) ±50% of the disk area with preretinal or vitreous hemorrhage

Macular edema (suggested by hard exudates within the macula)

Reduced vision from any cause

Immediate referral is strongly urged when the following are present.

Proliferative retinopathy less than high-risk characteristics

Preproliferative retinopathy with:

dilated irregular veins

cotton wool spots

multiple dot and blot hemorrhages

intraretinal microvascular abnormalities

Source: Reprinted with permission from Sperling, M. (Ed.). (1988.). *The physician's guide to insulin-dependent (type I) diabetes: Diagnosis and treatment* (p. 113). Copyright © 1988 by the American Diabetes Association, Inc.

tion, which is thought to be a factor in the cause of diabetic retinopathy (Early Treatment Diabetic Retinopathy Research Group, 1985). Use of a class of drugs called aldose reductase inhibitors is also being tried. By inhibiting aldose reductase, these drugs are thought to prevent the conversion of glucose to sorbitol and thereby prevent or slow the progression of diabetic retinopathy.

The effect of intensive insulin therapy in preventing retinopathy or slowing its progression is currently being evaluated.

Ophthalmologic Examination

Even though current treatment strategies cannot prevent or cure retinopathy, excellent evidence (Diabetic Retinopathy Study Research Group, 1979; Early Treatment Diabetic Retinopathy Research Group, 1985) suggests that they can

retard the progression of the disease if used appropriately and early in the course of the disorder. Therefore, careful evaluation of the eyes by primary care physicians and periodic referral to an ophthalmologist who specializes in the care of patients with diabetes are crucially important.

The Clinical Practice Recommendations of the ADA (1992, 1999; *Table 8-1*) state that a complete eye and visual examination by an eye doctor should be done at the time of diagnosis of diabetes and then at least annually in all patients more than 30 years old and in any patient 12–30 years old who has had diabetes for more than 5 years. The assessment should include examination with a slit lamp, measurement of intraocular pressure, and examination of the fundus after dilation of the pupil. Fundus photography is an excellent way to assess the retinal status. Fluorescein angiography is

TABLE 8-2

Visual Symptoms in Diabetic Patients That Require Further Evaluation and Treatment

Symptom	Possible Etiology	Management Strategy
Blurred vision	Poorly controlled Diabetes Mellitus	Control diabetes; no new glasses prescription for 4–6 wk
	Cataract Macular edema	Referral for comprehensive eye exam
Double vision	Diabetic mononeuropathy Other etiology	Neuroophthalmological and neurological evaluation; neurological referral frequently
Floaters	Vitreous hemorrhage Retinal detachment Retinal hole	Urgent referral for complete ocular evaluation
Ocular pain	Corneal abrasion Neovascular or angle-closure glaucoma Iritis	Emergency referral for complete ocular evaluation

Source: Reprinted with permission from Lebovitz, H. (Ed.). (1991). *Therapy for diabetes and related disorders* (p. 224). Copyright © 1991 by the American Diabetes Association, Inc.

used to check the patency of the retinal vessels and to find areas that may be contributing to macular edema.

Any patient who reports floating spots, flashing lights, or the sensation of having a curtain or veil in the visual field should be referred for immediate ophthalmologic attention. The patient may be having a vitreous hemorrhage, retinal detachment, or formation of a hole in the retina *(Table 8-2)*.

Other Ophthalmic Complications

Glaucoma

Glaucoma is a condition in which increased intraocular pressure has damaged the optic nerve and caused loss in the visual field. The frequency of glaucoma is slightly higher in persons with diabetes than for the general population. The prevalence of glaucoma increases with the patient's age and the duration of diabetes.

Open-angle glaucoma is 1.4 times more common in patients with diabetes than in people without the metabolic disorder (Aiello & Cavallerano, 1991). The outflow of aqueous humor in the eye is blocked, and the intraocular pressure increases. The patient has no symptoms; this is a painless type of

glaucoma. Timolol maleate or pilocarpine drops are used for treatment. An oral agent such as acetazolamide (Diamox®) to decrease production of aqueous humor may also be used. Argon-laser trabeculoplasty may be used to normalize intraocular pressure if medical therapy is ineffective.

Angle-closure glaucoma is a painful and acute condition in which the intraocular pressure is extremely high. Patients are very ill, have reddened eyes, and may be nauseated because of the pain. The intraocular pressure is lowered medically, and then surgery is done to create new outflow channels.

Neovascular glaucoma is more severe and sometimes occurs in patients who have severe diabetic retinopathy or retinal detachments or after cataract surgery. This type of glaucoma involves the growth of abnormal blood vessels, which impede the outflow of aqueous humor. Treatment, including medications, photocoagulation, and surgery, is not always successful. In some patients, the disease progresses to blindness and painful eyes. The treatment is alcohol injections for pain or enucleation.

Cataracts

Cataracts are opacities of the lens that occur commonly in the elderly. Cataracts tend to occur earlier and progress more rapidly in patients with diabetes than in people without diabetes. These opacities are 1.6 times (Aiello & Cavallerano, 1991) more common in patients with both type 1 and type 2 diabetes. The only treatment for cataracts is surgery, which is usually done on an outpatient basis.

Extraction of cataracts with and without a lens implant restores useful vision in about 90–95% of cases. Patients with proliferative retinopathy are at risk for the development of neovascular glaucoma, and intraocular lens implants are not used in these patients. For these patients, either contact lenses or cataract glasses (aphakic glasses) are used after lens removal.

Lens Changes

One of the first symptoms of diabetes experienced by many patients is blurring of vision. They often complain that their glasses are the wrong prescription. These changes occur because the lens of the eye swells in hyperglycemic states. Glucose on the lens of the eye is converted to sorbitol in the presence of aldose reductase, which is found in the lens, and results in osmotic changes and myopia at high blood glucose levels. Patients should be advised that the changes are temporary and that when blood glucose levels return to normal the symptoms will abate. Patients should not change prescription glasses until blood glucose levels have been stabilized for 4–6 weeks, because it takes some time for the lens to return to equilibrium.

Many patients report visual changes such as blurring, double vision, or bright flashing lights during episodes of hypoglycemia. These symptoms may be due in part to changes in the lens and a degree of cerebral edema (Ellenberg & Rifkin, 1983).

Ophthalmoplegia

Ophthalmoplegia are complications associated with neurologic changes and involve cranial nerves. Patients complain of double vision, which occurs because of paresis of one of the muscles innervated by the affected cranial nerve. Patients with involvement of the third cranial nerve may have some discomfort and drooping of the eyelid. Involvement of the fourth cranial nerve leads to double vision, and involvement of the sixth cranial nerve results in inward turning of the affected eye.

Episodes of ophthalmoplegia are distressing but usually resolve spontaneously in 4–6 months and require no treatment except support and adaptive measures. If an episode lasts longer than 6 months, the cause may not be diabetes, and further workup is required. Episodes may be recurrent and involve either the same or a different cranial nerve (Ellenberg & Rifkin, 1983).

NEUROPATHY

Diabetic neuropathy is the most common complication of diabetes. After 20 years of known duration of diabetes of either type, almost 50% of patients will have this complication (Pirart, 1977). In patients with type 1 diabetes, neuropathy usually does not occur within the first 5 years after diagnosis (Sperling, 1988). However, about 10% of in patients with type 2 diabetes have neuropathy at the time their diabetes is diagnosed. Both the incidence and the prevalence of neuropathy increase with the duration and severity of hyperglycemia.

Diabetic neuropathy involves a group of syndromes caused by damage to both the peripheral and the autonomic nerves as a result of the metabolic and vascular abnormalities of diabetes. Both the axon and the myelin sheath of the nerve are damaged, resulting in blockage of impulse transmission. Diabetic neuropathy is a form of "dying back" of the nerves in which the long nerve fibers are affected first. For example, symptoms first occur in the toes and later in the legs.

Diabetic neuropathies consist of many different syndromes, each with characteristic features and clinical courses. Because the syndromes overlap clinically and often occur simultaneously, no rigid system of classification has been adopted. Categories are often based on the type of nerve involvement, degree of vascular involvement, and the extent of nerve damage.

Diabetic Mononeuropathies

Mononeuropathies or focal neuropathies involve a single nerve or group of single nerves that are chronically exposed to pressure. The metabolic abnormalities of diabetes may make these nerves more susceptible to pressure. Symptoms include numbness, tingling, sudden onset of pain, and burning. The symptoms tend to be especially prominent at night.

Examples of mononeuropathies are carpal tunnel syndrome, third cranial nerve palsy-ptosis (see ophthalmologic complications), meralgia paresthetica, and footdrop (entrapment of peroneal nerve at the head of the fibula). Radiculopathy occurs when a spinal nerve root is affected, causing a loss of sensation and pain along the affected dermatome. Occasionally, patients with radiculopathy have abdominal pain.

Treatment of these neuropathies consists of recognition of nerve entrapment and correction. Pain is managed by splinting the affected area (e.g., the wrist in carpal tunnel syndrome) if possible, local injections of glucocorticoids to reduce swelling, and nerve block. Antiplatelet therapy (e.g., aspirin) is also sometimes beneficial. Prognosis is good, because mononeuropathies are curable, and spontaneous recovery often occurs within 3 months. However, if these conditions are left untreated, muscle weakness and wasting are likely to occur.

Proximal Motor Neuropathy

Examples of proximal motor neuropathy include diabetic amyotrophy and neuropathic cachexia. These are uncommon and usually occur in patients with mild type 2 diabetes and a long history of excessive alcohol intake. Signs and symptoms are asymmetric and include dramatic weight loss and a deep burning pain in the legs, pelvis, and thigh muscles. Patients have a loss of patellar reflexes, abnormal nerve conduction, and severe wasting of the quadriceps muscles.

Treatment includes analgesics, antidepressants, diet, strict blood glucose control, and physical therapy. Counseling to overcome alcohol abuse is essential. Recovery usually occurs in 2 years, with return of normal weight and relief of neuritic symptoms, but patients have some residual muscle weakness.

Distal Symmetric Sensorimotor Polyneuropathy

Distal symmetric polyneuropathy is the most common form of diabetic neuropathy. It is often called peripheral neuropathy, because it is characterized by an alteration of sensation beginning in the toes and fingers that progresses to the foot and hand in a "stocking-glove" manner. Symptoms are generally absent or mild in the initial stages but progress to numbness, tingling, burning, dull ache, and cramping that are worse at night and are relieved by arising and walking. Symptoms can progress to muscle weakness, sensory loss, unbalanced gait, foot ulcers, footdrop, and loss of fine motor skills.

Many patients remain free of symptoms, and in these cases, it is essential to carefully assess whether the patient has numbness or cold or "dead feet." Patients with chronic unrecognized neuropathy may not seek care until they have complications, such as foot ulcers, foreign objects embedded in the foot, unrecognized trauma to the extremities, or neuroarthropathy, associated with the later stages of peripheral neuropathy.

Neuroarthropathy (Charcot's joints) refers to joint erosions, unrecognized fractures, demineralization, and devitalization of bones that result from walking on a foot that has lost its normal proprioceptive and nociceptive functions because of neuropathy. In the most advanced stages of this condition, the radiographic appearance of the foot resembles that of a "bag of bones." All of these conditions are avoidable with proper early diagnosis and treatment of neuropathy.

Treatment for peripheral neuropathy is symptomatic, palliative, and supportive, with special emphasis on preventing the advanced-stage problems. Pain is managed with the use of analgesics and tricyclic antidepressants to allow the patient to rest at night. Capsaicin® cream applied topically is also used. Tight control of blood glucose levels is instituted, and improving the glycemic control may provide some relief of symptoms. Physical therapy is used in addition to muscle relaxants and nonsteroidal antiinflammatory drugs to relieve muscle pain.

Autonomic Neuropathy

Autonomic neuropathy involves the nerves that supply small blood vessels and sweat glands of the skin, the cardiovascular system, the gastrointestinal system, the genitourinary tract, and the adrenergic system. Autonomic neuropathy usually occurs in conjunction with distal symmetric polyneuropathy. Signs and symptoms are varied and depend on the system affected *(Table 8-3)*.

Cardiovascular autonomic neuropathy. The initial signs and symptoms of cardiovascular autonomic neuropathy (also called cardiac denervation syndrome) are due to involvement of the vagus nerve. This syndrome is manifested by a fixed heart rate of 80–90 beats per minute that does not respond to stress, mild exercise, sleep, or postural changes (Pfeifer,

---

TABLE 8-3
Syndromes of Autonomic Neuropathy

Cardiovascular autonomic neuropathy
> Resting sinus tachycardia without sinus arrhythmia (fixed heart rate)
> Exercise intolerance
> Painless myocardial infarction
> Orthostatic hypotension
> Sudden death

Gastrointestinal autonomic neuropathy
> Esophageal dysfunction
> Autonomic gastropathy and delayed gastric emptying
> Diabetic diarrhea
> Constipation
> Fecal incontinence

Genitourinary autonomic neuropathy
> Erectile impotence
> Retrograde ejaculation with infertility
> Bladder dysfunction

Hypoglycemic unawareness
Sudomotor neuropathy
> Facial sweating
> Heat intolerance
> "Gustatory" sweating

Source: Reprinted with permission from Sperling, M. (Ed.). (1988.). *The physician's guide to insulin-dependent (type I) diabetes: Diagnosis and treatment* (p. 127). Copyright © 1988 by the American Diabetes Association, Inc.

1991). As the dysfunction progresses, interference with normal cardiovascular reflexes, loss of exercise tolerance, a predisposition to orthostatic hypotension, tachyarrhythmias, "silent" or painless myocardial infarction, and sudden death occur.

Gastrointestinal autonomic neuropathy. Esophageal dysmotility can cause dysphagia, retrosternal discomfort, and heartburn. Gastroparesis (neuropathy of nerves supplying the stomach), or dilation and delayed emptying of the stomach, causes anorexia, nausea, vomiting, early satiety, and postprandial bloating and fullness. The delayed absorption of nutrients complicates control of blood glucose levels and produces unexplained swings between hyper-glycemia and hypoglycemia.

Diabetic gastroenteropathy, or neuropathy of the nerves of the small intestine, involves impairment in the intestinal fluid and elec-trolyte reabsorption and secretion. Signs and symptoms include severe, intermittent episodes of diarrhea that often alternate with constipa-tion. Diabetic diarrhea is typically incontinent and painless and occurs at night.

Genitourinary autonomic neuropathy. Impotence occurs frequently in men with dia-betes and is characterized by impairment of erectile function in the presence of normal libido. Other causes of impotence such as psy-chogenic, endocrine, vascular, and drug- or stress-related factors must be ruled out. Retrograde ejaculation, which may or may not occur with impotence causes infertility. Female patients may experience dyspareunia (painful intercourse) because of decreased vaginal lubrication and a diminished ability to experi-ence orgasms.

In the initial stages, neurogenic bladder is char-acterized by a diminished sensation of bladder fullness and reduced urinary frequency. These progress to incomplete emptying of the bladder and urinary retention with overflow inconti-nence and predispose the patient to urinary tract infections.

Autonomic sudomotor dysfunction. Signs and symptoms of autonomic sudomotor dysfunc-tion include excessive perspiration on the trunk and face with anhydrosis (lack of sweating) on the lower extremities. The dryness and crack-ing on the feet and legs can contribute to the development of ulcers. Functionally, there is a lack of ability to regulate the body core temper-ature, a situation that can lead to heat exhaus-tion or heat stroke.

Hypoglycemia unawareness. Lack of the usual warning signs and symptoms of hypoglycemia such as hunger, tachycardia, and diaphoresis leads to hypoglycemia unawareness. This con-dition is attributed to neuropathy of the adrenal medulla with a blunting of the adrenergic response to hypoglycemia (Sperling, 1988). This type of neuropathy predisposes patients to severe hypoglycemia and is a contraindication for rigid blood glucose control.

Treatment. Treatment of the autonomic neu-ropathies is sign and symptom specific. It is important to rule out other treatable causes of the signs and symptoms at the outset. The cor-nerstones of therapy are normalization of blood glucose levels, frequent blood glucose monitor-ing, and medications. Aldose reductase inhibitors are being evaluated as treatment. Because many of the neuropathies cause embarrassment and diminished self-esteem, support and understanding by the patient's family and the health care team are essential (see chapter 9).

Treatment of cardiovascular neuropathy includes instructions to the patients on appro-priate intensity of exercise, avoidance of hypo-glycemia (low concentrations of blood glucose can intensify cardiac irregularities), and avoid-ance of sudden positional changes. Accompanying orthostatic hypotension is man-aged by correcting hypovolemia with fluid replacement, improved glucose control, and increased sodium intake; elastic stockings; mineralocorticoids; vasoconstrictors; a military antigravity suit; or atrial pacing.

Treatment of gastrointestinal neuropathy is spe-cific to the signs and symptoms and includes small, frequent soft-to-liquid diets and the use of metoclopramide (Reglan®) for gastroparesis. A stool softener and a high-fiber diet are used in patients with constipation. For patients with diabetic diarrhea, medications such as broad-spectrum antibiotics and antispasmodics are used.

The delay in gastric emptying time and nutrient absorption often results in a mismatch between insulin peak action and blood glucose levels when insulin is given before meals. The time of insulin administration can be delayed to correct this mismatch and result in a correction in fluctuating blood glucose levels.

Management of urinary dysfunction includes scheduled voluntary urination, use of Credé's method, cholinergic-stimulating drugs, sphincter relaxants, and periodic catheterization. Surgical intervention may be required if these measures are ineffective, because chronic urinary retention may lead to infection, subsequent hydronephritis, and renal failure.

In men, impotence is often treated (after ruling out other causes) by appropriate counseling and surgical implantation of penile prostheses. Nonsurgical techniques involving vacuum devices, oral medications, and the injection of vasoactive drugs such as papaverine are also used. Management of female sexual dysfunction includes counseling and the use of vaginal creams to increase lubrication.

Treatment for sudomotor dysfunction includes avoidance of intense heat and education of the patient about ways to prevent heat stroke and hyperthermia. Skin and foot care is essential, with special emphasis on the use of emollients and proper footwear.

Patients with hypoglycemia unawareness must be taught to monitor blood glucose levels frequently. Realistic levels of blood glucose control that help avoid episodes of hypoglycemia should be individually determined for these patients.

NEPHROPATHY

Diabetes is the most common cause of nephropathy. Nephropathy is the most costly complication of diabetes due to the success of renal dialysis and kidney transplants. The earliest sign of this complication is albumin in the urine. Generally end stage renal disease occurs between 10 to 25 years duration of diabetes. One of four patients starting dialysis has diabetes (Sperling, 1988). African Americans, Hispanics and Native Americans all have greater prevalence of diabetic nephropathy than Caucasians with diabetes. In areas where the prevalence of type 2 diabetes is extremely high (e.g., areas with large populations of Pima Indians), more than 90% of the dialysis patients have diabetes.

Pathogenesis

The major functions of the kidneys are to (1) remove water, urea, creatinine, and other waste products to form urine; (2) maintain electrolyte and acid-base balance; (3) help maintain blood pressure; and (4) produce erythropoietin, a hormone that helps in the manufacture of red blood cells. The kidneys filter the entire blood supply every 2 minutes. The glomerular filtration rate is the rate at which the blood is filtered through the glomerulus. The normal rate is 125 ml/minute. The concentration of blood urea nitrogen is the blood level of urea, which is the end-product of protein metabolism. The normal concentration is 8–20 mg/dl and varies according to protein intake, state of hydration, and intake of steroids. Creatinine is formed from muscle metabolism, varies slightly with body size, and is normally 0.5–1.4 mg/dl.

Most patients with diabetes who have renal insufficiency have a history of poor glycemic control. Diabetic nephropathy has a genetic component and tends to occur repeatedly in families. Hemodynamic abnormalities, excessive protein intake, hypertension, metabolic abnormalities, neurogenic bladder, trauma, and toxic drugs or dyes are also causes of diabetic renal disease.

Progression

Type 1 Diabetes

At the time of diagnosis of type 1 diabetes, no renal histologic abnormalities are present, but renal blood flow and the glomerular filtration rate are higher than normal. When blood glucose levels are normalized, the glomerular filtration rate returns to normal. However, within 3 years, histologic changes of an increase in the amount of mesangial matrix material and thickening of the glomerular basement membrane occur.

Incipient diabetic nephropathy develops over the subsequent 10–15 years in about 30–40% of patients (DeFronzo, 1991). During this quiet stage, urinary excretion of albumin increases without clinically detectable proteinuria. Microalbuminuria, excretion of albumin at a rate of 25–250 mg/day, is the first laboratory evidence of diabetic renal disease that can be detected with newly available screening tests. Institution of tight glycemic control with insulin during this stage may prevent the development of diabetic neuropathy (DeFronzo, 1991).

Often, about 15 years after diagnosis of diabetes, clinically detectable proteinuria has developed (more than 250 mg/day), and the patient's long-term prognosis is guarded. The glomerular filtration rate may still be higher than normal at the onset of proteinuria, but it usually declines to about 50% within 3 years. This decline is an ominous sign and signals the onset of progressive renal insufficiency.

The concentrations of serum creatinine and blood urea nitrogen become higher than normal. Within approximately 2 years after the serum level of creatinine becomes elevated (more than 2.0 mg/dl), one half of the patients have progressed to end-stage renal failure. Uremia is defined as a glomerular filtration rate of less than 15 ml/minute.

Usually, patients with a serum creatinine level greater than 5 mg/dl cannot carry out normal activities because of the effects of uremia.

As the disease progresses, patients experience progressive signs and symptoms of uremia, beginning with anorexia and intermittent nausea, drowsiness, and lethargy. Anemia occurs because of diminished production of erythropoietin and more rapid death of red blood cells. Hypoglycemia occurs because of decreased degradation of insulin with decreasing filtration and the erratic oral intake due to nausea and anorexia. The dosage of insulin usually requires adjustment.

In addition, a myriad of other metabolic abnormalities occur, including hypoalbuminemia, hypovolemia, hyperkalemia, hypocalcemia, and increased serum levels of cholesterol and triglycerides. The signs and symptoms of complications involving the peripheral and autonomic nervous system are accentuated by the accumulation of toxins.

Type 2 Diabetes

In patients with type 2 diabetes, the course of diabetic nephropathy is less well defined. Albuminuria or microalbuminuria is usually present at time the diabetes is diagnosed. Racial background plays a larger role in type 2 diabetes than in type 1 (see introduction of this chapter). In most white patients, diabetic nephropathy does not progress to end-stage renal disease. When albuminuria is present in these patients, it is a predictor of death from stroke or myocardial infarction. Approximately 80% of these patients of cardiovascular complications die within 10 years.

Treatment

During Preclinical Period

Current evidence suggests that maintaining euglycemia may protect patients with diabetes from microvascular disease. Hypertension is the single most important factor that accelerates the progression of diabetic nephropathy. It also contributes to other causes of morbidity and mortality in patients with diabetes. Losing weight, reducing cholesterol and triglyceride levels, following a low sodium diet, and using diuretics are ways to control blood pressure. Recent studies suggest that angiotensin converting enzyme inhibitors and calcium channel blockers can be effective in treating hypertension.

Avoiding and treating urinary tract infections and avoiding the placement of an indwelling catheter (intermittent catheterization is less likely to introduce pathogens) are important measures to reduce kidney damage.

Patients should avoid the use of nephrotoxic drugs (e.g., aminoglycosides such as gentamicin) and nonsteroidal antiinflammatory agents such as ibuprofen and sulindac. Use of radiographic contrast agents should be avoided (particularly if the creatinine level is more that 3.0 mg/dl). If contrast material is necessary, mannitol given intravenously 1 hour before to the study offers some protection.

A low-protein diet (0.8 mg of protein per kilogram of body weight) (Powers, 1998) can slow the progression of renal disease. Dietary phosphate may also be restricted.

During Clinical Nephropathy

The treatment strategies used in the preclinical stage are continued during the stage of clinical nephropathy. Once end-stage renal failure begins, prolonging life requires dialysis or a renal transplant. These procedures should be discussed with the patient and the patient's family well in advance of this stage so that adequate planning can be done. Absolute indications for dialysis or transplantation include a concentration of serum creatinine higher than 8 mg/dl or a creatinine clearance rate of 10 ml/minute or less and severe signs and symptoms of uremia (Sperling, 1988).

Dialysis is the cleansing or filtering of the blood through a semipermeable membrane. During dialysis, the patient's blood passes on one side of the membrane, and the dialysate (prepared dialysis solution) passes on the other side. The dialysate draws fluid and waste products out of the blood.

Hemodialysis is the most common (about 80%) type of dialysis. Vascular access (often an arteriovenous shunt in the forearm) must be established and maintained. The treatment can be done at home, but it is often done at an ambulatory care facility. It is usually done three times a week for 4–6 hours each time.

Peritoneal dialysis is a process in which blood is filtered through the peritoneal membrane that lines the abdominal cavity. An intraperitoneal catheter is sewn in place. Patients and their families can learn to do this type of dialysis at home. Insulin, antibiotics, and other drugs can be added to the dialysate, freeing the patient from subcutaneous injections. Continuous ambulatory peritoneal dialysis is a manual method of peritoneal dialysis in which the patient exchanges the dialysis solution every 4–6 hours. Exchange of peritoneal dialysates has been simplified by use of a mechanical cycler. When the mechanical cycler, is used the procedure is called continuous cyclic peritoneal dialysis. With both continuous ambulatory and continuous cyclic peritoneal dialysis, patients are at constant risk for peritonitis (Davidson, J., 1986).

For kidney transplantation, a kidney from a living related donor, a living unrelated donor, or a suitable cadaveric donor can be used. Immunosuppressive medications are required throughout the patient's life to prevent rejection of the transplanted organ. Insulin requirements are increased after transplantation, because the newly functioning kidney catabolizes insulin again and posttransplant steroid therapy has a hyperglycemic effect. Combined transplantation of both kidney and pancreas is also done.

MACROVASCULAR COMPLICATIONS

Macrovascular complications of diabetes involve changes in the moderate- to large-sized arteries and veins. Unlike the case in microvascular disease, the known duration of type 2 diabetes does not seem to have a major effect on macrovascular complications. In type 1 diabetes, however, there appears to be a relationship between the age of the patient and the duration of diabetes in the development of these complications.

Atherosclerosis is a common change observed in diabetes and is literally a hardening in which mounds of lipid material mixed with smooth muscle cells and calcium accumulate in the inner walls of blood vessels. These formations are called plaques, and continue to grow, decreasing the diameter of the blood vessel. Eventually, the deposits or the formation of a blood clot along with diminished elasticity of the vessels causes a partial closure or an occlusion, and blood flow is interrupted.

There is a unique link between cardiovascular disease and type 2 diabetes or impaired fasting glucose. People with type 2 diabetes or IFG have abnormally high glucose levels, and along with hyperglycemia they are likely to have a group of other risk factors known as the "insulin resistance syndrome" or "Syndrome X." In spite of high levels of circulating insulin, the insulin is not able to overcome the hyperglycemic state, because of the inability of the cells to use the insulin effectively.

Clinical manifestations of Syndrome X include hyperglycemia, hyperinsulinemia, hypertension, dyslipedemias and increased levels of plasminogen activatior inhibitor-1 (PAI-1). The high levels of PAI-1 contribute to increased coagulation and clot formation. Dyslipidemias include decreased high density lipoproteins (HDL), elevated low-density lipoproteins (LDL), elevated very low-density lipoproteins (VLDL) and increased triglyceride levels. This cluster of risk factors helps to explain the high risk for complications and deaths from cardiovascular disease.

Macrovascular complications are more common, tend to occur at an earlier age, and are more severe and extensive in patients with diabetes than in people without diabetes. These complications contribute significantly to the morbidity and mortality of those who have diabetes.

Coronary Heart Disease

The risk factors for cardiovascular disease, which are the same for people with or without diabetes, are hyperlipidemia, hypertension, smoking, obesity, and a family history of heart disease. However, the overall incidence of cardiovascular disease is higher in the diabetic population.

Diabetes is an independent risk factor for atherosclerotic cardiovascular disease and increases the risk for this complication twofold to threefold. Women with diabetes are at particular risk and do not seem to have the normal "protection" of nondiabetic women. The rates of cardiovascular disease in women with diabetes, even before menopause, are several times those of women without diabetes and parallel the rates in men who have diabetes (Kannel & McGee, 1979).

Many studies indicate that coronary artery disease accounts for at least half the deaths in patients with diabetes. Patients with diabetes are more likely than people without diabetes to have an acute myocardial infarction at an earlier age and to have complications from that episode and to die of a myocardial infarction or to experience a second myocardial infarction.

As in people without diabetes, coronary heart disease is associated with chest pain, shortness of breath, and congestive heart failure. Patients with diabetes are more likely to experience a silent myocardial infarction without the typical signs and symptoms associated with ischemia, which may be due to autonomic neuropathy (see the section on autonomic neuropathy earlier in this chapter). Unexplained onset of congestive heart failure and the loss of blood glucose control to the point of diabetic ketoacidosis or hyperglycemic hyperosmolar nonketotic syndrome may indicate silent myocardial ischemia or a myocardial infarction.

Treatment of coronary heart disease is both medical and surgical. Medical treatment includes aspirin, nitrates, calcium channel blockers, antiarrhythmics, thrombolytic therapy, and antihypertensive agents. Surgical interventions include angioplasty and bypass surgery.

Cerebrovascular Disease

Patients with diabetes are also likely to have cerebral vascular disease at an earlier age than people without diabetes (Keen & Jarrett, 1979). This finding is true for both transient ischemic attacks and thrombotic cerebral vascular accidents. Studies have suggested that the mortality rates for both men and women with diabetes are three to five times greater than those of people without diabetes.

Signs and symptoms of cerebrovascular disease include intermittent dizziness, transient loss of vision, slurring of speech, paresthesia or weakness of one limb, and the occurrence of a stroke. Noninvasive techniques such as Doppler studies and scans are used to determine the diagnosis.

Treatment is aspirin or anticoagulants. Depending on the affected area, surgery may be considered.

Peripheral Vascular Disease

Peripheral vascular disease is common in patients with diabetes, especially those with type 2 diabetes (Levin, 1991). The incidence of occlusive peripheral arterial disease is approximately four times higher in diabetic men and six times higher in diabetic women than in those without diabetes (Keen & Jarrett, 1979). About half of all the lower extremity amputations done in the United States are on patients with diabetes.

Peripheral vascular disease is characterized by pain in the buttock, calf, or thigh that occurs during exercise and is relieved with rest (intermittent claudication). Additional signs include a cold foot or limb, shiny skin, thickened nail with fungus infection, discolored or blue mottled appearance, absence of hair, dependent rubor, decreased pulses, and presence of ulcers.

Treatment with Trental® (pentoxifylline), which decreases blood viscosity, lessens the signs and symptoms by increasing the blood flow. Other treatment include aspirin, a prescribed exercise program, and vascular surgery to open or bypass clogged vessels.

Risk Factors for Macrovascular Disease

Patients with diabetes have a number of risk factors for macrovascular complications (*Table 8-4*). Some factors are not preventable or treatable, such as age, genetic makeup, and duration of diabetes. However, several risk factors can be either eliminated or treated. Patients should be educated about these factors, because reduction of the factors has a great impact on both the development and course of complications.

Smoking

Smoking is the most important of the treatable risk factors (Levin, 1991). The smoking of one cigarette causes spasm of the arteries and reduces blood flow for approximately 1 hour. Smoking tobacco also decreases the level of serum high-density lipoprotein, increases platelet aggregation and the level of fibrinogen, and decreases erythrocyte flexibility.

Hypertension

Hypertension is much more common in patients with diabetes than in people without the metabolic disorder. Among patients with type 2 diabetes, 50% have hypertension as compared with

---

TABLE 8-4
Risk Factors for Diabetic
Macrovascular Disease

Nontreatable

    Genetic

    Age

    Duration of diabetes

Treatable

    Smoking

    Hypertension

    Hypercholesterolemia

    Hypertriglyceridemia

    Hyperglycemia

    Hyperinsulinemia

    Obesity

    Miscellaneous

        Inotropic drugs

        ß-Blockers

Source: Reprinted with permission from Lebovitz, H. (Ed.). (1991). *Therapy for diabetes and related disorders* (p. 329). Copyright © 1991 by the American Diabetes Association, Inc.

---

only 20% of people without diabetes (Levin, 1991). The risk of cardiovascular death in patients with diabetes is approximately doubled by the presence of hypertension (Sowers, 1991). Obesity is often associated with hypertension in patients with type 2 diabetes.

A first-line treatment of hypertension then is nutritional strategies. These include restriction of calories and weight loss, sodium restriction to 3,000 mg/day, restriction of alcohol intake, and regular exercise (ADA, 1992). Medications used to treat hypertension include calcium channel blockers, angiotensin converting enzyme inhibitors, and a- and ß-adrenergic blocking agents. ß-Blocking agents are used with caution, however, because of their tendency to cause hypoglycemia unawareness

and to interfere with both secretion of insulin and recovery from hypoglycemia (Sowers, 1991).

Hyperlipidemia

Hyperlipidemia occurs in 44% of patients with type 2 diabetes (Levin, 1991). In patients with diabetes, hyperlipidemia may be caused by poor metabolic control, associated conditions such as hypothyroidism, inborn errors of lipid metabolism, obesity, and poor dietary habits.

Nutritional strategies are fundamental in the overall management and prevention of lipid abnormalities in patients with diabetes. Other aspects are promotion of an exercise program, and establishment of good blood glucose control. If these measures are not successful in controlling lipid levels, five classes of hypolipidemic drugs are used: bile acid binding resins, nicotinic acid, fibric acid derivatives, hydroxymethylglutaryl-CoA reductase inhibitors, and probucol (ADA, 1992).

Hyperglycemia

Although associations between hyperglycemia and diabetic complications have been repeatedly shown for microvascular disease, such an association is weaker for macrovascular disease. The possible contributions of chronically elevated levels of blood glucose to the development of atherosclerotic vascular disease are as follows: With hyperglycemia, sorbitol accumulates in the intima of the blood vessel, where atherosclerotic plaques form. Protein glycosylation within the artery wall may contribute to atherosclerotic vascular disease. Increased fibrinogen levels are an independent risk factor for cardiovascular disease and correlate positively with blood glucose concentrations in both men and women (ADA, 1992). Treatment of hyperglycemia is necessary to eliminate signs and symptoms and to correct the associated lipid abnormalities.

Hyperinsulinemia

In people without diabetes, high levels of insulin in the bloodstream are associated with an increased risk of coronary artery disease. Some of the studies have shown that high levels of insulin may also be linked with atherosclerotic vascular disease in patients with type 2 diabetes. Treatment of hyperinsulinemia is directed at correcting the underlying cause of insulin resistance (need for more than 200 units/day), such as excess calorie consumption, obesity, and sedentary lifestyle.

THE DIABETIC FOOT

Amputation is a significant concern for most patients with diabetes. This concern is justified, because most major amputations (approximately 50% of lower extremity amputations) in the United States are done on patients with diabetes. Etiologic factors for diabetic foot include damage by external forces and pressures, thermal injury, chronic edema, obesity, and fungal or bacterial infections. Minor trauma leading to ulceration is the precipitating event for diabetic foot problems. The combination of neuropathy, vascular insufficiency, and an altered response to infection makes patients with diabetes especially susceptible to serious consequences of foot injury.

Neuropathic changes that occur in diabetes are sensory loss (dead feet) and the loss of position sense of the foot. Motor neuropathy affects all the muscles of the foot and leads to deformities such as protrusion of the balls of the feet (metatarsophalangeal joints), hammer toes, and arch elevation (pes cavus). The abnormal weight-bearing surfaces break down, and calluses and trophic ulcerations result. Autonomic neuropathy results in altered blood flow with a falsely warm foot. Anhydrosis or reduction in sweating leads to abnormally dry skin, which tends to develop cracks and fissures. Peripheral vascular disease with resultant chronic ischemia and an altered response to infection complete a triad that predisposes patients with diabetes to severe consequences.

Prevention

Educating patients about care of the foot is essential *(Table 8-5)*. In addition to wearing proper footwear and limiting foot pressures by other means, patients should examine their feet daily for fissures, cracks, hot spots, small suppurations, and ingrown nails. Instruction on skin and nail care and information on the criteria for and importance of seeking professional care for problems are also important.

Treatment

Treatment of the diabetic foot is best done by a podiatrist who is familiar with the particular needs of patients with diabetes. Self-treatment by patients is extremely dangerous and most often results in serious sequelae. When infections and ulcers occur, a variety of measures are used. The most important factors are "off-loading" pressure from the foot, adequate debridement, antibiotics to treat infections, proper dressings, and revascularization. Newer methods of treating ulcers include topical application of growth factors to improve healing.

CUTANEOUS DISORDERS

Skin disorders develop in 30% of patients with diabetes (Gilgor & Lazarus, 1981). Skin problems are often more of a problem in patients with diabetes than in those without and may require prompt and aggressive treatment to prevent the development of more serious complications. The underlying pathophysiology of the cutaneous disorders is not well understood.

Waxy Skin and Limited Joint Mobility

Up to 30% of patients 1–28 years old who have type 1 diabetes have limited mobility of the small and large joints. In patients who have had diabetes for more than 4.5 years, the severity of joint disease is correlated with microvascular complications (Bolognia & Braverman, 1991). The limited mobility is readily apparent: When the palmar surfaces of

---

TABLE 8-5
A Sample Foot-Care Teaching Session

- Have the patients remove their shoes and stockings. (Women can leave panty hose on.) Remove your own shoes and stockings along with them so that you can demonstrate procedures to the group.

- Demonstrate how to inspect shoes for proper fit. Explain that shoes that allow 1/2 to 3/4 inch of toe room are best. Suggest that patients with neuropathy who cannot feel for proper fit draw the outline of their feet on heavy paper, cut it out, and put it into shoes to test the fit.

- Suggest that they buy shoes in the middle of the day, when feet have swelled slightly, but not as much as they might by evening. Emphasize that they should be fitted for shoes by an experienced salesperson.

- Explain that shoes made of natural fibers, such as leather or canvas, are best because they breathe (allow perspiration to escape). Caution them against wearing thongs or plastic shoes and suggest that they be cautious about wearing sandals and walking in bare feet.

- Demonstrate feeling the inside of shoes for foreign objects, wrinkled insoles, and breaks in the shoes that might cause lesions. Suggest shaking shoes out before putting them on each time.

- Have the patients look at their stockings while you again discuss natural fibers. Stockings made of wool or of a high percentage of cotton also allow feet to breathe. Have them check that their stockings fit well and are free of darns or holes.

- Ask the members of the group to check their stockings to be sure that they do not compromise circulation. Remind them not to use tight-fitting garters or rubber bands to hold up their stockings. Panty hose, garter belts, or socks and knee-high stockings that have wide elastic bands will interfere less with blood flow. Pinch the stocking to assess for tightness. Suggest that they avoid sitting with legs crossed for long periods of time, and elevate their legs as an alternative position.

- Demonstrate how to perform a daily foot inspection. Look first for dryness or dampness. For dry feet, suggest a lotion that does not contain alcohol. For damp feet, suggest use of talcum powder. Tell them not to soak their feet; it can dry the skin.

- Have them look for areas of redness, corns, calluses, and lesions and suggest that those who have them be sure to get shoes that fit properly.

- Show the various products available for padding corns and bunions. Explain how corns and calluses can be softened and removed gradually with a pumice stone. Tell them never to cut them or use caustic products to remove them.

- Have the patients look for cracks and fissures and explain how they can become infected. Suggest treating unbroken cracks with an emollient.

- Ask each person to look at his own toenails. Demonstrate the proper technique for trimming them, using a volunteer. Suggest that they treat split or cracked nails with mineral oil. Advise those who have fungal infections, ingrown toenails, or planter warts to see a podiatrist and/or vascular surgeon as indicated.

- Show them how to pad overlapping toes with sheepskin or cotton.

- Pass around mirrors to demonstrate how each person can check the soles of the feet for calluses, corns, and ulcers. Suggest that those who have ulcers see a physician.

Source: Christensen, M., et al. (1991). How to care for the diabetic foot. *American Journal of Nursing, 91*(3), 52.

---

the hands are placed together, the palms and fingers do not lie flat against each other. About 35% of patients with limited joint mobility have tight, thick, waxy skin over the back of the hands that is difficult to tent. There is no treatment for this disorder. However, with improved blood glucose control, the cutaneous findings sometimes are reversed.

Scleredema

Scleredema is a thickening of the skin found most commonly on the upper part of the back and the posterior part of the neck. It may not be visu-ally apparent, but it sometimes develops a peau d'orange (orange peel) appearance. Less common sites include the face, upper arms, abdomen, lower back, and tongue. Patients are often unaware of these areas. There is no treatment. Some cases resolve spontaneously.

Diabetic Dermopathy

Diabetic dermopathy (shin spots) starts as multiple discrete, flat-topped, asymptomatic, dull-red papules 5–12 mm in diameter. The spots occur most often on the legs (knees to ankles) but may also occur on the forearms, thighs, and feet. Usually four or five lesions appear symmetrically over a period of a week. They may heal completely over several years, leaving a thin, hyperpigmented, slightly depressed area. New lesions continue to appear. These lesions cannot be induced by trauma, and there is no treatment (Gilgor & Lazarus, 1981).

Necrobiosis Lipoidica Diabeticorum

Necrobiosis lipoidica diabeticorum is an uncommon skin disorder that occurs in 0.1–0.3% of patients who have diabetes. It occurs almost exclusively in patients who have diabetes or in whom diabetes eventually develops. It is characterized by red to red-brown to violet plaques that enlarge and often become yellow in the center. The lesions appear most often on the shins. The lesions may ulcerate, especially after trauma, and are painful and slow to heal (Bolognia & Braverman, 1991). Treatment is aspirin, corticosteroids, and pentoxifylline.

Disseminated Granuloma Annulare

Disseminated granuloma annulare is characterized by many small, ringed lesions made up of individual plaques. The lesions are often on the trunk of the body. The skin in the center of the lesion may be normal in appearance or erythematous. Corticosteroids are used for treatment.

Xanthomas

Several types of cutaneous xanthomas are reflections of hypercholesterolemia and hypertriglyceridemia. The treatment consists of correcting poorly controlled diabetes with insulin. With better glucose control, the triglyceride levels decrease, and the xanthomas quickly resolve.

Acanthosis Nigricans

Acanthosis nigricans is characterized by velvety tan to dark-brown plaques on the sides of the neck, in the axillae, and in the groin. This skin disorder can be due to an underlying malignant neoplasm, but it is more commonly associated with

obesity and insulin resistance. Treatment includes weight loss, which reduces insulin resistance, and topical agents.

Bullosis Diabeticorum

Diabetic bullae are characterized by the rapid formation of serous blisters on the surface of the toes, feet, fingers, and forearms. The blister base is not inflamed, and there is no pain. The bullae usually occur in middle-aged to elderly patients who have a long history of diabetes. The lesions usually heal in a few weeks without scarring. Treatment consists of breaking the blisters, draining the fluid with gentle compression, and use of topical antibiotics.

PERIODONTAL DISEASE

Periodontal disease (also called pyorrhea) is a chronic, progressive bacterial infection that destroys the supporting tissues of the teeth. Patients with diabetes are especially prone to periodontal disease, and an exaggerated alveolar bone loss occurs in diabetic patients (Fritz & Offenbacher, 1986). Changes seen in the oral cavity of patients with high blood glucose levels include elevated calcium concentrations, elevated salivary glucose levels, higher levels of Candida albicans, and an alteration of oral microbial flora (Rosling, Slots & Genco, 1982).

Good dental hygiene, plaque removal, and mouth care are paramount for patients with diabetes. The use of fluoride helps inhibit tooth decay and may also help kill bacteria. The use of baking soda with hydrogen peroxide has been recommended for eradicating subgingival microflora (Villeneuve, Treitel & D'Eramo, 1985). Regular checkups and cleanings in addition to blood glucose control can drastically reduce periodontal disease. If surgery is necessary, prophylactic antibiotic therapy is often used.

EXAM QUESTIONS

CHAPTER 8
Questions 66–81

66. Which of the following complications accounts for half of the deaths in diabetes?

    a. Retinopathy
    b. Nephropathy
    c. Coronary artery disease
    d. Neuropathy

67. Which of the following is an early sign of kidney damage in patients with diabetes?

    a. Decrease in serum level of creatinine
    b. Increase in renal blood flow
    c. Microalbuminuria
    d. Thinning of the glomerular basement membrane

68. Which of the following is a major intervention used during the asymptomatic phase of diabetic renal disease?

    a. Creation of a fistula for dialysis
    b. Prescription of a high-fiber diet
    c. Prescription of a high-protein diet
    d. Normalization of blood pressure

69. Which of the following is an appropriate intervention if clinical kidney disease occurs in a patient who has diabetes?

    a. Educate the patient about dialysis and transplantation.
    b. Increase the insulin dose.
    c. Prescribe a high-protein diet.
    d. Prescribe immunosuppressive agents.

70. Open-angle glaucoma is characterized by which of the following?

    a. Abnormal growth of blood vessels on the surface of the iris.
    b. Severe pain, red eyes, and nausea.
    c. Decreased intraocular pressure.
    d. Impeded outflow of aqueous humor.

71. For a diabetic patient over age 30, without severe eye problems, an ophthalmologic examination should be performed how often?

    a. Every 6 months
    b. Every 12 months
    c. Every 2 years
    d. Every 5 years

72. Which of the following ophthalmologic disorders tends to develop at an earlier age in patients with diabetes than in people without diabetes?

    a. Presbyopia
    b. Cataracts
    c. Farsightedness
    d. Glaucoma

73. Which of the following is characteristic of diabetic autonomic neuropathy?

    a. Hypertension
    b. Increased gastric motility
    c. Decreased creatinine clearance
    d. Hypoglycemic unawareness

74. Sensorimotor neuropathy should be suspected if the feet of a patient with diabetes have which of the following?

    a. Very dry skin

    b. Charcot's joints

    c. Tingling of feet and toes

    d. Thick, ridged nails

75. Which of the following seems to be a major factor for development of diabetic retinopathy?

    a. Duration of diabetes

    b. Obesity

    c. Isometric exercise

    d. Cigarette smoking

76. Which of the following signs and symptoms would a nurse assess as indicating a sign of uremia ?

    a. Increase in appetite

    b. Anxiety

    c. Polycythemia

    d. Lethargy

77. What are the major macrovascular diseases that affect patients who have diabetes?

    a. Coronary artery disease, nephropathy, peripheral vascular disease

    b. Coronary artery disease, cerebral vascular disease, retinopathy

    c. Cerebral vascular disease, nephropathy, peripheral vascular disease

    d. Cerebral vascular disease, coronary artery disease, peripheral vascular disease

78. Which of the following is the best treatment for gastrointestinal signs and symptoms of neuropathy?

    a. Administration of laxatives

    b. Eating three large regular meals

    c. Symptom-specific treatment

    d. Use of corticosteroids

79. Which of the following is used to treat erectile dysfunction that is due to autonomic neuropathy and is causing impotence?

    a. Cholinergic-stimulating drugs

    b. Weekly injections of estrogen

    c. Angiotensin converting enzyme inhibitors

    d. Surgical implants

80. Risk factors for development of macrovascular disease include which of the following?

    a. Decreased plasma levels of fibrinogen

    b. Hypolipidemia

    c. Controlled hypertension

    d. Obesity

81. Which of the following is a major point to be made during instruction on diabetes foot care?

    a. Neuropathic pain will eventually subside

    b. Careful, daily inspection of the feet and shoes is imperative

    c. The feet should be soaked for 2 hours daily

    d. Pain is a reliable indicator of any problems

CHAPTER 9

PSYCHOSOCIAL ISSUES

CHAPTER OBJECTIVE

After completing this chapter, the reader will be able to discuss how support systems, stress, and other psychosocial factors affect patients with diabetes and their families.

LEARNING OBJECTIVES

After studying this chapter, the reader will be able to:

1. Specify stress management techniques.

2. Recognize factors that influence the emotional response to diabetes by patients and their families.

3. Recognize the impact of diabetes on patients and their families.

4. Recognize the characteristics of the stages of adjustment involved in adapting to a chronic illness.

5. Specify the characteristics of adaptive and maladaptive coping to diabetes.

6. Indicate strategies to increase patients' adherence to diabetes management.

7. Specify resources beneficial to diabetic patients and their families.

INTRODUCTION

The development of the chronic condition of diabetes at any age disrupts the lifestyle of the patient and the patient's family. Life will never be quite the same. The unrelenting demands of diabetes do not go away after the acute symptoms present at diagnosis are resolved. Daily attention and tasks are required; patients are never again "free" of diabetes; it is always there.

Lurking in the background is the uncertainty of the future. Patients wait for the proverbial bombshell to explode, and questions abound. Will there be complications? Will I be disabled? How long will I live? How does this affect my family? Can I even have children? In addition, patients must simultaneously try to manage the usual person- and age-specific concerns of life. Many changes and adjustments are needed.

Stress has both a direct physiologic affect and an indirect impact on patients with diabetes. The support of a knowledgeable health care team and referral to appropriate resources can enhance patients' ability to "live well" with diabetes.

STRESS AND DIABETES

It is not clear what role stress plays in the onset of diabetes; however, stress clearly influences the course of the disorder (Ellenberg & Rifkin, 1983; *Figure 9-1)*. Several mechanisms by which

FIGURE 9-1 Interactions Between Psychological Stress and Glycemic Control

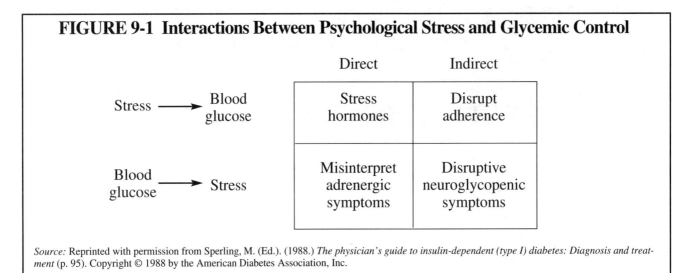

	Direct	Indirect
Stress → Blood glucose	Stress hormones	Disrupt adherence
Blood glucose → Stress	Misinterpret adrenergic symptoms	Disruptive neuroglycopenic symptoms

Source: Reprinted with permission from Sperling, M. (Ed.). (1988.) *The physician's guide to insulin-dependent (type I) diabetes: Diagnosis and treatment* (p. 95). Copyright © 1988 by the American Diabetes Association, Inc.

stress affects diabetes may coexist. (1) Altered emotional states are accompanied by hormone secretion patterns. (2) Stressful times lead to changes in diet intake, exercise, medications, and monitoring. (3) During stressful times, metabolically active agents such as alcohol and nonprescribed drugs may be used to deal with emotions.

Hormonal Responses

The body's response to stress is described as the general adaptation syndrome (Selye, 1957). The alarm reaction represents acute stress, the so-called fight-or-flight reaction. This response involves the sympathetic nervous system. The counterregulatory hormones epinephrine and norepinephrine are released into the bloodstream and cause a increase in blood glucose levels. If activity is greatly increased in this stage, severe episodes of hypoglycemia may occur.

The stage of resistance is the stage of chronic stress, in which elevated levels of cortisol cause glucose levels to remain high or become more unstable, resulting in difficulty in maintaining diabetes control. The stage of exhaustion marks the end of life or the manifestation of the full disease process.

Other Manifestations

Aspects of self-care may deteriorate when stress occurs. It may become more difficult to carry out the needed management activities of monitoring, medications, diet, and hygiene. Patients may forget to take their insulin, measure the dose incorrectly, eat too little or too much, and exercise more or less than normal.

Patients may confuse the adrenergic signs and symptoms of stress such as palpitations and sweating with those of hypoglycemia. They may compensate by overtreating for low blood glucose levels, causing a worsening of diabetes control. The signs and symptoms of true low blood glucose levels, which may occur, can be disruptive in work and social settings and can then increase stress. Some patients react to stress by using alcohol or nonprescribed or illegal drugs. These agents have a direct effect on physiologic reactions and affect the ability or desire to carry out diabetes management.

Assessing Patients for Stress

Patients need to understand how stress can affect diabetes, both the direct physiologic effects and the indirect impact it can have on diabetes control and well-being. A health care professional should assess patients' total adaptation to diabetes at each visit and be sensitive to any data that suggests stress. A well-structured interview should be conducted to elicit information about stressors such as lack of social support, lack of tension relievers such as hobbies and leisure time activities, and poor dietary or exercise practices. Recurrent health problems related to diabetes control such as repeated episodes of hypoglycemia, frequent recurrences of diabetic ketoacidosis, high levels of glycohemoglobin, and particularly unstable or "brittle" diabetes are objective indications that a patient likely has problems adjusting to diabetes.

If stress is suspected, several specific objective tools can be used to determine the source and degree of stress. These include the Holmes and Rahe Social Readjustment Rating Scale, Jaffee's Stress Map, and Sullivan's Diabetes Adjustment Scale.

Stress Management Techniques

An effective stress management plan should include good nutrition, an exercise program, a specific method to improve attitude, and information on techniques to reduce stress. Good nutrition includes following a well-balanced meal plan and, if needed, reducing the calorie level to attain desirable body weight (see chapter 2). Exercise should be regular and aerobic (see chapter 3).

Cognitive Restructuring

Use of cognitive restructuring techniques can help patients take a new perspective on a chronic problem such as diabetes and thus improve their lifestyle. Several different techniques can be effective.

Assertiveness training. Assertiveness training uses education, role playing, and other techniques to teach people how to act and converse in a nonaggressive yet assertive manner. Learning to be assertive with family members, friends, and health professionals promotes a sense of self-ownership of the control over management of diabetes.

Empowerment training. Empowerment training teaches patients ways to own and take control of life situations. Diabetes engenders a feeling of loss of control in patients. The techniques

learned in empowerment training allow them to regain the feeling of power over life situations.

Problem solving. Problem solving is a proactive stance that encourages people to assess a difficult situation, plan for intervening, implement the intervention, and then assess and refine the intervention for the future. It can be used on a daily basis to work on incremental steps to reinstitute control of diabetes management.

Time management skills. Learning time management skills can help with the problem of scheduling the tasks needed for good diabetes management. Learning to schedule time for both the planned management tasks and for work and recreational activities can help patients achieve a balanced lifestyle.

Other techniques. Self-talk involves using positive affirmations and thoughts to improve diabetes care, particularly when feeling overwhelmed by self-care tasks. Thought stopping is learning to say stop to defeating thoughts when they occur. Reframing is the process of turning negative thoughts or statements into positive ones. An example would be changing the statement or reframing "I hate pricking my finger for blood tests" into "Pricking my finger for blood tests may hurt a little, but the results let me know how much insulin I need so I can safely play my soccer game."

Stress Reduction Techniques

Biofeedback. Biofeedback is a method of determining the effectiveness of a technique used for relaxation or stress reduction. Biofeedback can be any process that gives information indicating a change in internal physiology. The change can be monitored by checking pulse rate, temperature, blood glucose levels, or blood pressure. Biofeedback can also involve equipment to measure muscle activity or brain wave activity.

Relaxation training. Relaxation training can be as simple as teaching deep abdominal breathing to be used as a strategy to relieve immediate stress. Progressive relaxation involves the conscious contraction and relaxation of muscles in a systematic process while focusing on this process and ignoring external stimuli. Relaxation can be used at any time and in any place. Several studies have shown that relaxation actually lowers blood glucose levels (Cox, Taylor, Nowacek, Holley-Wilcox & Pohl, 1984; Lammers, Naliboff & Straatmeyer, 1984; Rosenbaum, 1983).

Additional techniques. Other techniques can also be used to promote stress reduction. Imagery uses visualizing and focusing on pleasant scenes and memories for a "time-out" from problems. Meditation uses focusing on a sound, thought, or object to provide time away from daily stress. Music therapy promotes relaxation through the tune and tempo of music. Color therapy promotes relaxation through focus on progressively muted colors.

Participation in hobbies, sports, or other leisure time activities can be an effective method of stress reduction. People with diabetes and their families often have fears about sports activities and need information and even counseling to overcome these apprehensions.

THE EVOLVING PHASES OF DIABETES

From a psychological point of view, the course of diabetes has three major phases (Holmes, 1986).

The Diagnosis Phase

This first phase occurs immediately after diagnosis and lasts about a year. The focus is on learning about diabetes and adjusting to living with the diagnosis and adjusting to the required changes in lifestyle. This is a time for emotional adjustment for both the patient and the patient's family. Typically, this phase includes the evolvement through the stages of grief (which are discussed in a following section).

During the diagnosis phase, easy accessibility to and strong consistent support of health care providers are important for both the patient and the patient's family. At the beginning, emotions are high and interfere with the assimilation of the tremendous amount of new information that must be learned. Experts advise that only the most basic information (e.g., survival skills) be taught at the time of diagnosis to avoid overload and to allow time for working through the necessary psychological issues. As time progresses, patients and their families should be taught the skills and information necessary for living optimally with diabetes.

If the diagnosis phase is not resolved within a year, it is a warning signal that inadequate adjustment is being made and an indication that professional psychological help may be needed (Sperling, 1988).

The Maintenance Phase

The maintenance or midphase begins when the patient and the patient's family have learned to live with the diabetes and lasts until the onset of chronic complications. The primary task of this phase is developing and maintaining a workable plan for managing diabetes. The maintenance phase usually lasts several years and is often a period of well-being and full functioning.

The Complication Phase

The last phase is associated with the development of complications such as retinopathy, circulatory difficulties, and renal failure. During this phase, the grief process occurs again, this time over serious losses in health status such as blindness, amputation, dialysis, and impotence. Feelings of anger and despair are common. The multiple emotional reactions that come in the complication phase must be dealt with, and some resolution must be achieved before patients can come to a level of psychosocial equilibrium. Despite these obstacles, many patients and their families and significant others are able to make good adjustments to the patients' altered lifestyles.

REACTIONS TO THE DIAGNOSIS AND LOSS OF HEALTH

Patients and their families react in a variety of ways to the numerous challenges that a diagnosis of diabetes brings. A loss has truly occurred; the status of good health has been lost. Health care professionals who acknowledge and understand the mechanisms behind these reactions can act as a catalyst to help patients and patients' families achieve balanced outcomes.

Factors That Influence the Emotional Response to Diabetes

The type and intensity of emotional responses to diabetes depend on several factors *(Table 9-1)*. Some of these are age and stage of maturity at the time of diagnosis, basic personality, self-image, health care beliefs, and social and economic influences.

Age at Time of Diagnosis

In a child or younger person, a diagnosis of diabetes calls attention to the patient's mortality for the first time and presents new and totally unexpected obstacles. Patients can no longer coast along in well-established routines and react spontaneously. Living with diabetes requires not only changes in routines but also planning. Peers are of paramount importance in childhood and youth, and diabetes can severely affect those relationships and the attendant activities.

Generally, children's responsibility for self-care should increase with their cognitive, motor, and psychological development, beginning about the time they begin school. Active participation is important. It confers ownership on the child and results in better adherence to diabetes management.

Family tension can occur around the member who has diabetes. Healthy siblings can feel neglected as parents focus attention on the child with diabetes. Marital and family conflicts can arise, and even child abuse can occur. The best outcomes occur when a child with diabetes is treated as part of the family and the diabetes is considered just one of the special characteristics of that child.

TABLE 9-1

Factors That Cause Emotional Distress in Response to the Diagnosis of Diabetes

Uncertainty about the outcome of the immediate situation

Feelings of intense guilt or anger or both about the occurrence of diabetes

Feelings of incompetence and helplessness about the responsibility for management of the illness

Fears about future complications and early death

Loss of valued life goals and aspirations because of illness

Anxiety about planning for an uncertain future

Recognition of the necessity for a permanent change in living pattern due to diabetes

Source: Reprinted with permission from Sperling, M. (Ed.). (1988.) *The physician's guide to insulin-dependent (type I) diabetes: Diagnosis and treatment* (p. 91). Copyright © 1988 by the American Diabetes Association, Inc.

Hormonal changes, a focus on body image, and the tasks of attaining independence and establishing a career are issues important to successful passage through adolescence. The spontaneity of adolescence, particularly in regard to eating and activity, often directly conflicts with the treatment regimen for diabetes. Adolescents sometimes deliberately manipulate the regimen (e.g., use less insulin to lose weight, provoke episodes of diabetic ketoacidosis). Issues of smoking, substance abuse, and sexual freedom also complicate diabetes care during this stage of life.

If diabetes occurs during adulthood, marriage and family, employment, finances, planning for the future, and the anticipation of complications are some of the major concerns. Persons who have established independence must now deal with being in a more dependent role. The patient's spouse or significant other should become a full care partner in diabetes management.

In the elderly, a diagnosis of diabetes and the changes necessary for management can add overwhelming stress. These patients may already be somewhat isolated socially, have lost a spouse, and have some physical impairments.

Basic Personality Traits, Self-Image, and Health Care Beliefs

There is no "diabetic personality." Patients tend to react to diabetes in their usual pattern of response to a problem according to their personality traits, their self-image, and their beliefs about health. Patients who are independent tend to assume responsibility early and fully and gain independence in managing diabetes. Those who have been more dependent before the diagnosis often attempt to have families, spouses, or health care professionals be responsible for diabetes management.

A poor self-image before diagnosis adds one more negative in the patient's eyes to an already damaged self-image. Patients who have an intact and healthy self-image usually assimilate the diagnosis into their composite of self and function effectively.

A variety of health care beliefs exist in our culture, and these affect the individual response to the diagnosis (*Table 9-2*). Some people believe that treatment of a disease has little benefit and that no matter what is done, the end result will be the same. Others may think that the adverse effects on lifestyle dictated by following the management regimen (e.g., diet, exercise) far outweigh any possible benefits. Still others may believe that health care professionals overreact and impose unnecessary restrictions on lifestyles. These patients may state that they knew others who had the same diagnosis and without any care had no ill effects.

Common Initial Reactions at the Time of Diagnosis

Fear and anxiety. Fear and anxiety are common reactions to the diagnosis of diabetes. The statistics about diabetes or examples of people with diabetes who have had poor outcomes may produce fear. Often patients recall the experiences of a relative who had a difficult time with diabetes. Even though the relative's situation has no similarity to the present situation, the memory of the relative's problems has an adverse influence on the patient's perception of his or her own condition. A patient and his or her family may sit in the examining room cringing at the thought that the patient is in imminent danger of blindness, amputation, and kidney failure.

The anxiety that can result from this kind of fear can be destructive to self-care and the quality of life. Because of the fear, patients and their families may panic and freeze, becoming unable to perform even the simplest tasks needed for diabetes management. If unresolved, anxiety can become all-consuming and extend beyond the diagnosis of diabetes itself. It can affect relationships with family and coworkers.

TABLE 9-2
Health Care Beliefs Related to Diabetes

The patient's emotional response to diagnosis and treatment of Diabetes Mellitus and willingness to follow prescribed therapy depend in large measure on health-care beliefs.

To enhance success with prescribed therapy, the clinician should determine the patient's health-care beliefs and try to correct misconceptions before outlining the therapeutic plan.

It is important to determine the patient's attitudes about:

Susceptibility to the disease

Possible response (denial): "I hear what you are saying, but no one in my family has diabetes and I feel great. The laboratory probably made a mistake."

Consequences of the disease

Possible response (indifference): "I hear what you are saying, but so what? My dad has diabetes, and he's just fine. I feel great."

Value of treatment

Possible response (futility): "I believe you, but nothing can be done about the disease. I have a relative with diabetes who tried hard and did just what the doctor told him to do. He had a heart attack anyway."

Risks vs benefits of treatment

Possible response (defeat): "I believe that I have the disease, but what you are telling me to do will ruin my life. Isn't there another way?"

Source: Reprinted with permission from Rifkin, H. (Ed.). (1985). *The physician's guide to noninsulin-dependent (type II) diabetes: Diagnosis and treatment* (p. 56). Copyright © 1985 by the American Diabetes Association, Inc.

Some patients surrender to their fear and anxiety and live a life of defeat, incapable of functioning effectively. If filled with fears of possible complications, parents of young people with diabetes can become overprotective. This overprotectiveness can in turn lead to rebellion in the patient and not only worsen the diabetes management but destroy family relationships.

Fear and anxiety are poor motivators for improving self-care. Health care providers should not use examples of patients with severe complications. Most often, these examples terrify patients with newly diagnosed diabetes and result in panic or denial.

Guilt. Guilt is also a common response to the diagnosis of diabetes, especially when the patient is a child. Parents must realize that they cannot control the traits they pass to their children. Often husbands or wives blame each other's side of the family for bringing diabetes to the child.

Guilt is also a part of the response when people "moralize" about diabetes. It is important to avoid using terms such as "good blood sugars" and "bad tests." Terms such as "normal blood sugars" or "high tests" are less emotionally charged and judgmental.

Somatization. Somatization with the development of physical signs and symptoms such as diarrhea, vague abdominal complaints, headaches, and anorexia may appear. This reaction complicates the picture inordinately and is difficult to assess and manage.

Confusion. An overwhelming confusion also sometimes results when the diagnosis of diabetes is made. Confusion is especially common in older patients. Because of the impact of hearing the diagnosis, they simply cannot assimilate or integrate the information being presented.

Relief. Some patients and families initially experience a sense of relief at the diagnosis of diabetes. This reaction often occurs in patients who may have suspected that something they consider a worse diagnosis (e.g., cancer or AIDS) was the problem causing their signs and symptoms. Sometimes, when children start taking insulin and feel so much better, they express relief (and deep fears) that they are not "really going to die."

The Stages of Grief

It is quite common for both patients and families to experience grief when the diagnosis of diabetes is made. Feelings of loss are usually what sets this process in motion. Patients often feel a loss of control, a loss of "normal" functioning, and, most of all, a loss of freedom. The stages of grief associated with a chronic illness are modeled on the stages of adaptation to a diagnosis of terminal illness described by Elizabeth Kubler-Ross in her famous book *On Death and Dying* (1970).

Adapting to chronic illness is defined as working through the stages sequentially. However, the stages do not always occur for each person in a predictable order, and each stage does not last a predictable length of time. Some people may get "frozen" in a stage. Many people will go back and forth between the stages of adaptation and may experience some stages several times.

Denial. Denial is usually the first reaction. This is a state in which the person subconsciously behaves as if the unwanted circumstance (e.g., diagnosis of diabetes) does not really exist. Denial is a common and probably necessary protective or defense mechanism. At first it may be beneficial in easing the pain associated with the reality of having diabetes. A typical statement by a patient expressing denial would be, "I hear what you are saying, but there must be a mistake, because no one in my family has diabetes. I feel great. The laboratory probably made a mistake." Many patients with diabetes use partial denial by following only a part of needed management. For example, they may take their insulin but not follow a meal plan.

Unfortunately, if denial continues, it can be a large problem if it prevents patients from providing the care required for treatment of diabetes. Helping patients and families face denial is an important way that others can provide support. Education and group experiences with other patients and families are often helpful mechanisms for breaking patterns of denial.

Anger. Anger may be directed outward at family, friends, the health care team, or anyone who is "healthy" and does not have diabetes. Patients who had slight elevations in blood glucose levels for some time before complications developed are often angry with their physicians for "not telling me I had this terrible disease and now look what's happened to me." These patients fail to acknowledge that the physician has struggled with their denial for years.

Anger may also be directed inwardly. A patient might express it by asking, "Why did I eat so much sugar?" or "Why didn't I lose weight?" Anger is often a clue that a person has underlying feelings of frustration, fear, guilt, embarrassment, or inadequacy.

Bargaining. Bargaining may be a difficult stage to recognize. During this stage, promises are made "to do all those things (e.g., shots and tests) and do them just right" in exchange for the disease going away or a cure being found. The bargain may even be a subconscious one with a Supreme Being or the physician. This is a time when the outward attitude toward the diabetes is usually compliant and matter-of-fact. When the anticipated "payoff" does not occur, patients or their families become discouraged, and diabetes management often deteriorates.

Depression. When the full impact of the diagnosis is felt and the loss can no longer be delayed, depression occurs. Even though it is an expected occurrence, depression can have serious consequences. The symptoms of depression include tiredness, lethargy, irritability, sleep disturbances, change in eating patterns, decrease in activity, feeling alone and worthless, feelings of helplessness and hopelessness, and suicidal ideation or attempts.

The metabolic aberrations of poor diabetes control, especially prolonged hyperglycemia, can cause or contribute to these symptoms. Therefore the first step in lifting this depression is regaining blood glucose control and treating any physical problems. Depression can have serious outcomes for the patient and should be assessed and treated immediately. Referral to appropriate specialists may be indicated.

Acceptance or adaptation. The final stage is acceptance or adaptation. This stage is the optimal stage for patients and their families to reach in which they recognize and accept the responsibility of working with the health care team for optimal management of diabetes. Unfortunately, once reached, this stage is not permanent. Acceptance is a tenuous state that is often assaulted by the occurrence of complications, other health issues, and life stresses.

Impact of Diabetes on the Individual

The impact of living with diabetes varies greatly from person to person. For some, diabetes presents only minor difficulties. Others experience diabetes as an all-consuming and overwhelming burden.

It is impossible for persons without diabetes to understand the demands placed on a patient who has this disorder. Daily routines of insulin administration, blood glucose monitoring, dietary manipulations, and treatment of hypoglycemia take much time and effort.

Recreation and leisure activities are affected. Patients must plan and think about when and where they will eat. Activities that involve expending physical energy require decision making and planning to avoid extremes of blood glucose. Supplies must be packed and carried. There is no vacation from diabetes, it must be taken into account with every activity.

Two areas of major concern for many patients are employment and driving. Most jobs are available to persons with diabetes. Employers who have had a bad experience with a diabetic employee in the past may fear hiring or continuing to employ persons who have diabetes. *The Position Statement of the ADA* (1995) states, "Any person with diabetes, whether insulin dependent or non-insulin dependent, should be eligible for any employment for which he/she is otherwise qualified." Some occupations, such as being a member of the U.S. military, an airplane pilot, or an interstate truck driver, remain closed to patients with diabetes if insulin management is required. Guidelines of the Occupational Safety and Health Administration also limit the machinery in construction and factory work that a person with diabetes can operate.

The Americans with Disabilities Act of 1990, which became effective on July 26, 1992, offers protections in the workplace for patients with diabetes (Betschart, 1992). This act provides for the reasonable accommodation by employers for persons who have a disability. For patients with diabetes, this includes protections against discrimination in hiring and the need for the employer to accommodate individual schedules for meals and needed appointments.

Getting and keeping a driver's license can become an issue for people with diabetes. Some states now require a physician's statement attesting to diabetes control before they will issue or renew a driver's license. Physicians and other health professionals are required by law to report to the motor vehicle department any episode of hypoglycemia that involves loss of consciousness.

Coping with Diabetes

The degree of coping and the style of coping with diabetes varies greatly from person to person. As previously mentioned, several factors influence whether the coping is adaptive or maladaptive. These include personality characteristics, health beliefs, degree of stress and ability to manage stress, and available resources.

Adaptive Coping

Adaptive coping occurs when the grief process is negotiated in a healthy manner. The patient (or family member, in the case of children and the elderly) identifies himself or herself as the person responsible for the management of diabetes and makes a commitment to the treatment regimen. This commitment includes developing and using self-care skills to manage diabetes effectively.

Patients who cope well usually have an established support system, including family, friends, diabetes-related resources, and health care professionals, that they use well. In addition, these patients tend to participate in continuing education presentations, read diabetes-related periodicals, and attempt to stay informed of the trends and developments in diabetes care.

Maladaptive Coping

Maladaptive coping can take several forms. If a patient cannot progress through the grief process he or she can become stagnant and fail to function effectively. Failure to take responsibility for self-

care is the most obvious manifestation of maladaptive coping. Patients who ignore their diabetes plan or only perform the most minimal care (e.g., take enough insulin to avoid diabetic ketoacidosis); avoid medical care; or use defense mechanisms such as rationalization, repression, regression, withdrawal, and denial exhibit maladaptive coping styles.

Behavior modification techniques are sometimes effective in helping people improve when coping is maladaptive. Positive behavior modification that uses rewards for desired behavior may be effective in shaping improved behaviors in diabetes management (e.g., weight loss, regular monitoring of blood glucose level). Negative behavior modification involves the use of punishment or loss of privileges and is more controversial.

The Effects of Diabetes on the Family

Studies of patients with diabetes and their families have implicated a relationship between family functioning and diabetes control. Therefore, the adjustment that a family makes to the diagnosis of diabetes in one of its members takes on significant importance. The family needs resources for support just as the patient does. It is important that all family members learn about diabetes and have an opportunity to express and work through their feelings. Open communication becomes vital so that problems can be solved before they interfere with family dynamics and the patient's care.

Adaptive coping in the family is characterized by involvement in the educational process and diabetes regimen. Family members need reassurance about the patient and the disease. It is important for the family to achieve a balance between showing concern without being overanxious and promoting optimal diabetes care without being judgmental.

Maladaptive family coping usually takes one of two forms. A family member may distance himself or herself or be nonsupportive. He or she may also "sabotage" the patient's efforts (e.g., baking sweet desserts) or put obstacles to diabetes management in the patient's path. Another maladaptive coping form for families is to become overprotective and foster dependency on the part of the patient.

The presence of complications may have a severe effect on the family and patient with diabetes. Impotence is a complication that affects both the patient and the patient's spouse. Often sexual functioning is incompletely assessed, and the problem remains hidden and untreated, causing tremendous family stress. It is crucial for health professionals to determine if impotence exists and to direct the patient and his family to help. Other complications, such as retinopathy, nephropathy, and macrovascular complications, that result in restricted functioning also stress family relationships. Referral to appropriate resources may help alleviate these stressors.

ADHERENCE TO DIABETES MANAGEMENT

As many as one third to one half of all patients with diabetes do not adhere to their established plan of management for diabetes care. The list of possible barriers to adherence is virtually endless. Only a few are discussed here. Health care professionals must recognize the importance of eliciting information about barriers to adherence and then work with the patient and the patient's family to construct a plan of action to overcome these barriers and improve diabetes management.

Barriers

Barriers to adherence with diabetes management include the following:

- **Degree of life changes and the complexity of the diabetes management regimen.** If the changes are big or the regimen is complex or not understood well, the chances that the plan will fail increase.

- **Cost of care.** Diabetes is an expensive disease. The supplies may not be covered by insurance, and enough money may not be available for even the basic necessities. Consequently, patients may not monitor their blood glucose levels because they cannot afford the test strips and may refuse to attend classes to learn about diabetes.

- **Cultural factors.** In some societies, diabetes is considered a reflection of a curse on a family. Native Americans believe that it is an offense to refuse food offered when they are guests. Some Hispanics think that using insulin is dangerous and that herbs can cure diabetes.

- **Lack of support systems.** Patients who feel alone or unloved may not adhere to their management plan. They may not have assistance or transportation to attend classes or appointments.

- **Other stressors.** Events such as death in the family, loss or change in job, the threat of loss of job if diabetes is known, divorce, and illness of other family members also affect adherence.

- **Lack of knowledge or contradictory health beliefs.** If a patient and his or her family do not have a good understanding of diabetes and its treatment, adherence will be poor. If the health belief system (discussed earlier in this chapter) is in opposition to the regimen, the chances of adherence are almost negligible.

- **Poor self-image, feelings of defeat and powerlessness, and defense mechanisms.** Psychological factors may lead to attitudes of "What's the use?" or "Why try; its hopeless" or "I'm not worth all this effort."

- **Fears.** Fears, especially of hypoglycemia and loss of control, are extremely powerful in preventing patients and their families from attempting to gain normal blood glucose levels.

Strategies to Increase Adherence

Health care professionals can use several effective tools to increase adherence to the diabetes management regimen:

- **Encourage patients and their families to "take charge" of the diabetes management.** Taking over the lead in the health care of diabetes empowers patients and families.

- **Simplify the regimen within the bounds of appropriate diabetes management.** Patients and their families should participate in creating a plan of care that maximizes outcomes while simplifying the complexity of the tasks of caring for diabetes.

- **Focus on the normal, not the differences.** Help the patient be a person who sees diabetes as just one part of his or her total being.

- **Teach the tools and help the patient get supplies.** Teach patients and their families how to use tools such as blood glucose monitoring to better manage diabetes and assist them in obtaining supplies by referring them to resources for financial assistance when needed.

- **Provide a safe harbor.** Persons with diabetes and their families need a reliable and safe place on which they can rely. Health professionals can provide this place. Referral to support resources is an equally important service.

- **Provide adequate education and information.** Help patients and their families get the knowledge and skills they need to provide optimal care.

RESOURCES FOR PATIENTS AND THEIR FAMILIES

A wide variety of resources are available to help patients and families cope with diabetes (see also the appendix). Many times the resource may exist, but the person in need is not aware of it. Health care professionals can serve as the most important resource of all by maintaining current knowledge of resources and assisting patients and families in making contact with the most appropriate source of help and support. The following is a sample of the resources available.

Financial Resources

Insurance coverage is extremely important for patients who have diabetes. Currently, the most cost-effective type of private insurance is group coverage. Individual coverage can be obtained, and the local ADA maintains current lists of insurers who provide coverage for patients with diabetes. Some states are attempting to implement a pooled risk program for those who remain uninsured. Coverage for supplies, diabetes education, and medical care varies greatly. The best resource for obtaining coverage for supplies is to use a pharmacy that specializes in handling diabetes supplies and knows how to obtain reimbursement. Medicare and Medicaid are also important resources, and patients should be assisted in applying for these as needed.

Community food banks can sometimes help provide staples for patients in need. The Women, Infant and Children's Program helps supply food for pregnant women and young children. The Salvation Army or American Red Cross can be contacted for emergency financial assistance. Many hospitals have a fund that can be contacted for help with medications and supplies. Housing for families from out of town may be available through a Ronald McDonald House. Local charitable organizations such as Elks, Optimists, and so forth may help on a temporary basis to obtain assistive devices such as glasses or special foot wear.

Support and Educational Resources

The ADA offers many services, including the One to One Program (matches patients with newly diagnosed diabetes with patients who are successfully managing diabetes), support groups for adolescents and adults, diabetes camps for children and adolescents, educational programs, brochures and pamphlets, magazines and information, and referrals. The Juvenile Diabetes Foundation focuses on fund raising activities to find a cure for diabetes. The foundation provides information on the latest research, support groups for children and parents, a magazine, brochures and pamphlets, information, and referrals.

Many hospitals have diabetes educational programs and diabetes care centers. Classes are often at low cost, and scholarships may be available.

Other educational resources include a radio program, "Living with Diabetes," that is broadcast in several states; the Diabetes Control Division of the Centers for Disease Control and Prevention; the National Diabetes Advisory Board; the National Diabetes Information Clearinghouse; and the American Association of Diabetes Educators. Newsletters and magazines are available from many of these organizations. In addition, many of the companies that market diabetes supplies offer magazines, newsletters, and informational brochures on request.

Many specialized support groups and organizations, such as Insulin Pumpers Groups, also are available. They may supply materials in large print, audiotapes, and radio reading stations for visually impaired people.

Vocational Resources

Vocational rehabilitation needs can often be met through the state vocational rehabilitation agency. This agency usually can provide vocational counseling, job training, and job placement. Issues involving legal rights can often be addressed by the local Legal Aid Society.

Counseling Resources

Counseling can sometimes be obtained through the county mental health department. Ministers or hospital chaplains can also be important resources. The health care team should include a psychosocial health professional (psychologist, social worker, or counselor).

EXAM QUESTIONS

CHAPTER 9
Questions 82–90

82. A family's adaptive reaction to diabetes in a family member would include which of the following?

    a. Involvement in the diabetes regimen and realistic expectations

    b. Taking over the care for the patient

    c. Creating situations that hamper management goals

    d. Free expression of the burdens of caring for the patient

83. The adjustment process for a person with newly diagnosed diabetes is similar to the stages of adjustment to a terminal illness as defined by Kubler-Ross. Which of the following statements best characterizes this process in a chronic disease?

    a. The stages are experienced in a predictable order.

    b. The stages alternate and may be experienced several times.

    c. Once a stage has been experienced, it does not recur.

    d. People progress through the stages naturally and do not "get stuck" in any one stage.

84. A pilot with newly diagnosed type 1 diabetes should be referred to which of the following community resources?

    a. United Way

    b. Legal services

    c. Vocational rehabilitation

    d. None; having diabetes will not interfere with his license

85. Progressive relaxation consists of which of the following?

    a. Reframing

    b. Positive behavior modification

    c. Contraction and relaxation of muscle groups

    d. Problem-solving skills

86. A patient with newly diagnosed diabetes states, "I might as well be dead. I'll never be able to lead a normal life again." Which of the following would be the nurse's best response?

    a. After I teach you everything you need to know, you'll find out you're wrong.

    b. You will have to do some things differently to control this disease, but you can still lead a normal life.

    c. The doctor prescribed insulin, and this will take care of everything.

    d. Don't worry. Stress can affect your diabetes. Everything will be fine.

87. Coping strategies are most successful when a person has which of the following?

    a. An adequate support system

    b. Adequate time to practice

    c. Type 2 diabetes

    d. No complications

88. Diabetes may adversely affect a patient's personal relationships in which of the following ways?

    a. It prohibits following religious practices.

    b. It increases fears of rejection and abandonment.

    c. It prohibits obtaining a driver's license.

    d. It necessitates dietary measures that are detrimental to family members.

89. Adequate adjustment to having diabetes may be evidenced by which of the following behaviors?

    a. Repeatedly losing diabetes identification

    b. Refusal to see medical personnel

    c. Attending initial diabetes classes and all updates offered

    d. Allowing family members to take the major responsibility for care

90. Which of the following statements about the health beliefs of a person with diabetes is correct?

    a. Their beliefs must always be changed to accommodate treatment for diabetes.

    b. Their beliefs never prevent compliance with physicians' orders.

    c. Their beliefs are easily changed once teaching-learning occurs.

    d. Their beliefs affect the response to the diagnosis of diabetes.

CHAPTER 10

USING THE NURSING PROCESS IN THE CARE OF PATIENTS WITH DIABETES MELLITUS

CHAPTER OBJECTIVE

After completing this chapter, the reader will be able to utilize the knowledge gained in the previous chapters to the application of the nursing process in caring for patients with Diabetes Mellitus.

LEARNING OBJECTIVES

After studying this chapter, the reader will be able to:

1. Specify the four components of the nursing process.

2. Indicate factors that affect learning by adults.

3. Select appropriate examples of using the nursing process in the care of patients with diabetes.

4. Apply knowledge of diabetes learned in previous chapters to case studies.

INTRODUCTION

The nursing process determines the way nurses structure and guide their practice. Little and Carnevali (1976) define the concept in their book on nursing care planning, stating that the nursing care process "labels a concept involving a pattern of observations and logical thinking that is the basis for formulating the nursing care plan." The nursing process is really problem solving applied to the care of patients. It provides an organized, deliberate, and systematic approach to practicing the art and science of nursing.

The nursing process is dynamic and continual and not static. Its use requires constant attention and updating. It forms a basis for communication within the nursing professions and with other health care providers, patients, and patients' families. It also provides a structured approach to facilitate patients' involvement in care and parallels the self-care process that patients and their families are practicing simultaneously.

Nursing is carried out in a variety of settings within the health care delivery system. Nurses are one part of the health care team that works with the patient and the patient's family to manage diabetes. Because of the expanding scope of nursing practice, nurses on the health care team must have expert skills in interviewing and gathering data, carrying out observation and assessment, practicing new clinical techniques, understanding the pathophysiologic and psychological processes, and coordinating resources to optimize care.

THE NURSING PROCESS

The nursing process consists of four separate but interrelated components: assessment, planning, implementation, and evaluation. These components are discussed individually, and case discussions are used to illustrate the application of the previously presented material to the particular step of the process and the nursing process as a whole.

Certain issues, although not a specifically named step in the nursing process, are vital to successful interactions with patients and their families. Some of these issues (Yura & Walsh, 1978) are as follows:

1. A degree of trust must be established between the patient and the patient's family and the nurse.

2. A definition of roles must occur in the relationship between the patient, the patient's family, and the nurse.

3. An opportunity must be given for the participants to voice fears, raise questions, and begin to feel comfort in their roles.

4. An environment must be established that fosters full participation.

The degree to which these issues are successfully dealt with influences the success of the pursuit of the nursing process.

Successful use of the nursing care process with patients who have diabetes demands that the nurse also be familiar with and a proponent of patient self-care. These skills are valuable in helping patients and their families assume effective daily management of diabetes.

ASSESSMENT

Assessment, the first step in the nursing process, is essential in determining the areas that require intervention. It should be an orderly process that determines the problems and concerns of a patient so that a plan of care and management can be formulated. Assessment may be done through direct observation; a structured interview; casual conversations; written information such as charts, reports, and clinical data; and interactions with other members of the health care team.

Assessment of a patient with diabetes should focus on the whole person; that is, it should be done from a holistic perspective. Therefore, it is not limited to the patient's initial physical or emotional problem. Instead, it includes the patient's and the patient's family's perception of the problem as well as objective data.

Determining the patient's current health practices, such as dietary intake, smoking, use of alcohol, exercise, compliance with previously determined diabetes management regimens, and health care beliefs will allow incorporation of these individual practices into the management plan. The assessment should include data on risk factors associated with diabetes as well as the actual presence of complications, other health problems, and treatment.

In addition to gathering information on the physical and emotional parameters of the patient and the patient's family, the nurse must assess their knowledge base and learning needs. Assessment of learning needs involves obtaining information about the patient's readiness and capacity for learning, manual dexterity, visual acuity, social history, family support, and other variables that may affect the outcome of the educational process. This assessment can provide a realistic picture to both patients and their families and the health care team of the potential for self-care and the extent of family involvement or outside resources needed.

Assessment data should be recorded as a part of the patient's permanent record. Sharing this information with other members of the health care team is essential. After the assessment data are collected, the nurse analyzes this information and determines the problems, actual or potential, for which intervention is needed. Assessment is ongoing, and the problem list may change as new data are collected.

Case Example 1

Joe Black, 58-year-old man with type 2 diabetes, was admitted to the hospital 4 days ago for treatment of a foot ulcer. Mr. Black has had diabetes for 8 years and takes Glucotrol® (glipizide) at home. He reports that although his blood glucose levels "are not perfect," he has little problem with his diabetes.

In the hospital, he is not taking Glucotrol; he is receiving sliding-scale insulin to maintain blood glucose control. The teaching house staff is making rounds and asks for input on Mr. Black's blood glucose readings. The nurse reports the following objective data:

> At bedtime last evening Mr. Black's blood glucose reading was 123 mg/dl. This morning, Mr. Black's blood glucose concentration is 311 mg/dl. He reports that he slept very poorly last night and states that he had "horrible dreams" during the night and has a headache today.

Questions

1. What is happening to this patient to cause his concentration of blood glucose to be so erratic?

2. What assessment data could the nurse gather to help define the problem?

3. What knowledge can be helpful in assessing and analyzing that data?

Discussion

In carrying out an assessment, the nurse gathered some important data in this case that helped in devising an improved plan of care for the patient. The written orders for blood glucose monitoring for this patient specified checks of blood glucose level three times a day and at bedtime and treatment with sliding-scale insulin. The orders were transcribed as follows: Check blood glucose levels and give sliding-scale insulin at 8 a.m., 12 noon, 6 p.m., and 8 p.m.

However, because meals on this particular nursing unit were served at 7 a.m., 11 a.m., and 5 p.m., the checks were all of postprandial levels. Therefore, insulin was being given after the patient had eaten, not before as the prescribing physician intended. The orders were changed to read as follows: Check blood glucose levels before meals and give sliding-scale insulin. On the basis of the patient's reported symptoms and knowledge of insulin action times, the nurse recognized that the patient was probably having a hypoglycemic reaction in the middle of the night. The nurse reported her assessment to the physician, and the next day the care plan was changed so that the sliding-scale insulin was held at bedtime despite a concentration of blood glucose of 256 mg/dl at that time. (This patient has type 2 diabetes, so some insulin is being produced.) The patient woke the next morning with a blood glucose concentration of 168 mg/dl and stated he had slept very well. The nurse also determined that the patient had been treated with an excessive amount of simple carbohydrate for hypoglycemia. She made plans for in-service teaching for the other nurses on the unit about treatment of hypoglycemia.

PLANNING

The care plan is an action plan that incorporates the determined needs or problems, the proposed approaches of intervention, and methods to evaluate the effectiveness of the interventions. Included in the plan are outcome goals with behavioral objectives. The goals may be short, intermediate, or long term. They must, however, be realistic and measurable. The plan must also be flexible, because conditions change, and the unexpected can occur.

Ideally, the planning is a group activity that involves all the members of the health care team, community resources, the patient, and the patient's family. The ultimate goal is to help patients help themselves. If the plan is oriented in terms of the patient's expectations, goals, and capabilities, the chances for success are increased. The input of the patient's family is crucial in supporting the plan and the patient in carrying out the plan both directly and indirectly. A knowledge of resources and methods of referral can be valuable in ensuring that the plan can be implemented.

All patients with diabetes should be assessed for their educational needs, and these needs should always be included in the plan and care of the patient. The ADA (1999) lists 15 content areas that are to be included in the educational plan:

1. General facts about diabetes

2. Psychological adjustment

3. Family involvement

4. Nutrition

5. Exercise

6. Medications

7. Relationship between nutrition, exercise, and medications

8. Monitoring

9. Hyperglycemia and hypoglycemia

10. Illness

11. Complications (prevent, treat, rehabilitate)

12. Hygiene

13. Benefits and responsibilities of care

14. Use of health care systems

15. Community resources

An important component of the planning phase is the setting of measurable behavioral objectives. The best behavioral objectives consist of the following:

1. Who will do an action

2. What the action will be

3. When the action will be done

4. The extent or quantity to which the action will be done

Case Example 2

Susan Jerome, a 17-year-old with type 1 diabetes, was admitted to the nursing unit at 4 a.m. after 2 days of lethargy, polyuria, polydipsia, and uncontrollable vomiting. She has lost 6 pounds (2.7 kg) in the past week. About 5 days before admission, she had flulike signs and symptoms. Her appetite was poor, and when she started vomiting, her mother decided not to give her insulin because of limited food intake. At admission, Ms. Jerome's blood glucose concentration was 465 mg/dl, and a test for ketones in the urine was 3+. She was given insulin by drip for diabetic ketoacidosis and normal saline for hydration.

Ms. Jerome responded quickly to treatment. By 6 p.m. her blood glucose level was 130 mg/dl, and she asked for something "solid" to eat, because she had tolerated the sodas and snacks she had in the midafternoon. The insulin drip was discontinued at 7 p.m. after she had eaten dinner, and sliding-scale insulin was ordered to be given before meals. At midnight, the night nurse who was making rounds noticed a peculiar "sweet odor" at Ms. Jerome's bedside. Ms. Jerome was very lethargic and difficult to arouse. Fingerstick glucose monitoring indicated a glucose concentration of 342 mg/dl.

Questions

1. What has happened to this patient and why?

2. What kind of planning should have been done to prevent this from happening?

3. What kind of plan should be made for educating Ms. Jerome and her mother?

Discussion

The patient has most likely gone back into diabetic ketoacidosis. Several things were missed in planning care of this patient who had diabetic acidosis at the time of admission. Her blood glucose level should have been monitored often enough during the time she was being treated with the insulin infusion to note when the concentration of blood glucose had decreased to 250 mg/dl. At that time, the physician should have been notified and most likely would have changed the fluid infusion to dextrose to allow for the presence of sufficient glucose to provide nourishment.

When an insulin infusion is discontinued, little insulin is circulating after 15–20 minutes, so it is necessary for the nurse to plan to administer subcutaneous insulin before the infusion is discontinued. Without this dose of insulin, patients with type 1 diabetes cannot use the glucose available (see chapter 7 for a full discussion).

The physician's order, which was written when the insulin drip was discontinued, was for sliding-scale insulin to be given before meals. However, because the patient had already eaten by the time the insulin infusion was discontinued, administration of sliding-scale insulin was scheduled to begin at breakfast the next morning.

With good assessment skills, including knowledge of physiology, to help in planning, the nurse could have requested an order for subcutaneous insulin to be injected before the insulin infusion was discontinued. An example of an objective of the nursing plan of care would be as follows: The patient will receive adequate insulin to prevent a reoccurrence of diabetic ketoacidosis during this hospitalization.

In planning for the educational needs for this patient and her mother, it is clear that a review of sick day management is needed and an understanding of why insulin is needed even when dietary intake is diminished. The report indicated that the patient's mother, not the patient herself (17 years old), decided not to give the insulin. An assessment of the situation may indicate that planning is needed to help this patient be more independent in the management of her diabetes. The following are

examples of some of the educational objectives for her:

- Before discharge from the hospital, the patient will be able to explain why insulin is always needed even if oral intake is diminished.

- Before discharge from the hospital, the patient will be able to list 10 examples of fluids and foods to be used on sick days in place of foods on the normal diet.

IMPLEMENTATION

Implementation refers to carrying out a plan of care. It includes all the nursing activities and all the activities of the patient and the patient's family that help the patient meet the determined needs and solve the problems that have occurred. The patient's family and significant others should be actively involved whenever possible. They can provide support and reinforcement during the action phase and cues for appropriate behavior by the patient.

Many of the procedures that involve care of diabetes in the acute care setting must also be carried out after the patient is discharged from the health care facility. It is crucial to foster the patient's independence in the hospital setting and allow for supervised practice of these procedures (e.g., glucose monitoring and insulin administration).

Several techniques to enhance learning come from the writing of the "father of adult education," Malcolm Knowles. Learning occurs optimally under the following circumstances:

- The learner feels a need to know what is being taught.

- The material is related to what the learner already knows.

- The material being taught is personally relevant to the learner.

- The information or skill can be applied immediately and repeatedly.

- Opportunities for practice and rehearsal are given.

- The learner is given feedback.

- The learner has confidence in his or her ability to actually perform the behavior being taught.

With patients of any age, it is important to remember that education about diabetes and its management should be staged. Thus, survival skills are taught first during the initial or acute phase after the diagnosis. This phase is followed by a more comprehensive course in the self-management of diabetes. Finally, a plan is made for update and review and the addition of advanced topics such as lifestyle flexibility and special situations (e.g., carbohydrate counting, insulin adjustments).

Case Example 3

Guy Shrock is a 65-year-old man with insulin-requiring type 2 diabetes who was referred to the diabetes center for outpatient evaluation and education. He is 5 feet 11 inches (180 cm) and weighs 192 pounds (86.4 kg). He states that he has lost about 5 pounds (2.25 kg) in the past 3 months. At this time, he is taking 100 units of NPH insulin at bedtime daily, and the usual range of his blood glucose level is 350–450 mg/dl. He has severe leg pain and a "dead feeling" in his feet and fingers. He had cataract surgery on his right eye about a month ago and says, "I can see perfect with it now." Surgery for cataract extraction for the other eye is planned.

This is Mr. Shrock's second referral to the diabetes center. He received education 2 years before this visit when he was being started on insulin therapy (15 units) because oral antidiabetic agents did not provide adequate blood glucose control. At that time, he was taught how to monitor his blood glucose levels with a glucose meter obtained for him through Medicaid. He was also given instruction by the dietitian about an 1,800-calorie ADA diet,

and an exercise plan was made with him that called for walking 30 minutes/day.

Mr. Shrock brought his Accu-Chek III® to the visit. It was calibrated incorrectly, and according to the expiration date on the vial of strips of a different code number, the strips were no longer good. He said that he really had not used the meter very much because he could not "quite remember the steps you told me." He also brought his vial of NPH insulin. It was newly opened, did not have any clumping, and mixed well.

Questions

1. What kinds of problems could be occurring with this patient?

2. What interventions would be most effective for this patient?

3. When a plan is made, how can it best be implemented?

Discussion

During the assessment, the nurse asked Mr. Shrock to show how he drew up the insulin. He completed drawing up the injection and stated that it was ready. The syringe contained only 20 units of insulin, and the plunger was on the 100-unit mark. These findings were pointed out to him, and he was instructed to fill the syringe again. This time when he was finished the syringe contained approximately 10 units of insulin although the plunger had been pulled down to the 100-unit mark. He was given a magnifying device (Magni-guide®) to attach to the syringe, and he was able to correctly draw up a full 100 units of insulin. In order to assess the impact of this dose, he was sent home with two predrawn syringes that he correctly prepared. At the return visit 3 days later, his fasting blood glucose level was 168 mg/dl.

The nurse also determined that Mr. Shrock could not deal with the complexity of his glucose meter. A new meter was obtained through Medicare, because he was now 65 years old. He was instructed in the use of this simpler meter which required no coding or timing and was able to perform monitoring without a problem.

At the second visit, Mr. Shrock saw the dietitian to review his dietary intake. He revealed that he was drinking a lot of juice for his fruit servings. The dietitian reviewed the exchanges with him, and Mr. Shrock agreed to limit juices and use whole fruit. He was given a newly available booklet with pictures of food choices that he stated "makes it much easier to figure out what I'm supposed to eat."

In order to ensure that the implementation of the plan was complete, a referral to home health services was made to help Mr. Shrock in his daily environment. Follow-up showed that he was able to decrease his insulin dosage to 25 units daily, with blood glucose in the range of 135–160 mg/dl, and that his neuropathy symptoms had improved so much that he was able to walk 20–30 minutes/day.

EVALUATION

The final phase of the nursing process is evaluation. How effective is the diabetes management? Success is measured by the achievement of objectives that are mutually determined by the health care team and the patient and the patient's family. Failure to achieve these objectives necessitates a reassessment of the patient, a determination of why the goals were not met. The nurse can ask questions such as the following: Were there problems such as failures in communication, unrecognized complications, lack of support, lack of follow-up, lack of knowledge or understanding, or inappropriate tools or referrals? The answers to these queries can be useful in developing a new and revised plan of care.

Case Example 4

Josephine Barnett is a 73-year-old patient who has had diabetes for 17 years. She has been admit-ted to the unit for treatment of a leg ulcer. Before the admission, she had been taking 15 units of NPH insulin before breakfast and dinner. Now she is being given sliding-scale regular insulin before meals. When the nurse measured the concentration of Mrs. Barnett's blood glucose before lunch, it was 215 mg/dl. The nurse administered 6 units of regular insulin according to the sliding scale as was ordered. Mrs. Barnett ate her lunch about 20 minutes later. Forty-five minutes later, her roommate called the nurse to the room and stated that Mrs. Barnett needed a nurse immediately. Mrs. Barnett was lying on the bed. She was diaphoretic with cool skin, complained of a headache, and was very upset. She said, "I'm just so shaky. Something is wrong with me."

Questions

1. What has happened to this patient?

2. What should the nurse do for this patient?

Discussion

The patient has the classic signs and symptoms of hypoglycemia. The nurse should give Mrs. Barnett some fast-acting source of simple carbohydrate, according to protocol, and check her blood glucose level. Because the nurse had correctly planned care and implemented care, there is a need to evaluate why the plan of care was not successful.

Evaluation

The nurse began evaluating the plan of care by reviewing Mrs. Barnett's chart. A similar episode had occurred on three other occasions during this hospitalization. Each time, Mrs. Barnett's blood glucose reading has been high enough before a meal to require insulin and about 1.0–1.5 hours after her meal, Mrs. Barnett had similar signs and symptoms of a low blood glucose level, but felt better after treatment. During Mrs. Barnett's interview about her management at home, she mentioned that she really did not eat big meals because she always felt so full and distended after eating.

Questions

1. What kind of an evaluation can be made of the physiologic responses of the patient?

2. On the basis of the evaluation, how can the nursing care process improve the patient's care?

Discussion

The nurse used assessment skills by obtaining both objective and subjective data. She checked the chart and interviewed Mrs. Barnett because she suspected that Mrs. Barnett might have gastroparesis. After the nurse discussed her findings with the other members of the health team and with Mrs. Barnett, the nursing care plan was changed so that Mrs. Barnett's insulin was injected about 30 minutes after her meal. This change resulted in improved blood glucose levels and eliminated the hypoglycemic events.

EXAM QUESTIONS

CHAPTER 10
Questions 91–98

91. Under what circumstances does an adult patient with diabetes learn optimally?

    a. The patient's blood glucose level is elevated.

    b. Discharge from the hospital is imminent.

    c. The nurse explains in detail why change is necessary.

    d. The patient is given an opportunity for practice.

92. What are the four steps in the nursing process?

    a. Analysis, preparation, intervention, and education

    b. Assessment, planning, implementation, and evaluation

    c. Analysis, planning, intervention, and evaluation

    d. Assessment, preparation, intervention, and evaluation

93. Which of the following concepts is important in educating a patient with type 1 diabetes?

    a. Take oral antidiabetes medications with meals.

    b. Use of urine glucose testing tablets.

    c. Always take insulin.

    d. Call the doctor if you develop headaches.

94. For hospitalized patients on sliding scale insulin, blood sugars should be checked

    a. every six hours.

    b. two hours after meals.

    c. every four hours.

    d. before meals.

95. Symptoms of gastroparesis include

    a. hunger immediately after eating.

    b. postprandial bloating and fullness.

    c. nightmares.

    d. albuminuria.

96. Effective behavioral objectives specify

    a. when the action will be done.

    b. the laboratory results.

    c. the name of the hospital.

    d. the admission date of the patient.

97. A nurse plans the care of an obese patient with newly diagnosed type 2 diabetes on the basis of knowledge that therapy will focus on which of the following?

    a. Starting insulin immediately.

    b. Starting one of the oral hypoglycemic agents immediately.

    c. Maintaining adequate body weight.

    d. Planning the diet, adding oral hypo-glycemic agents if needed, and using insulin if oral agents do not work.

98. Which of the following might be anticipated in the nursing assessment of a diabetic patient receiving a sulfonylurea who has a severe infection?

    a. The infection cannot be effectively treated until the sulfonylurea is discontinued.

    b. Insulin may be needed to control the level of blood glucose.

    c. The dose of the sulfonylurea will need to be reduced.

    d. The signs and symptoms of the infection will be masked.

CHAPTER 11

FUTURE HORIZONS IN DIABETES MANAGEMENT

CHAPTER OBJECTIVE

After completing this chapter, the reader will be able to discuss current areas of research in diabetes.

LEARNING OBJECTIVES

After studying this chapter, the reader will be able to:

1. Specify two methods of noninvasive blood glucose monitoring that are being investigated.

2. Indicate the importance of autoimmunity in the development of type 1 diabetes and emerging methods of early treatment for this disorder.

3. Recognize three areas of research in the treatment of diabetes.

4. Indicate the advantages of the implantable insulin pump.

INTRODUCTION

Diabetic patients and their families and friends all anxiously await the results of research that can cure or lessen the impact of diabetes on daily life and the lifelong manifestations of this disease. Researchers all over the world are investigating the cause of diabetes and are seeking a cure. They are also developing devices and products to help patients maintain better diabetes control.

Research on type 1 diabetes is centered on pancreas transplantation, the development of an artificial pancreas with a closed or feed-back loop, development of an implantable pump, and the prevention of diabetes. Work on type 2 diabetes is focused on the causes of obesity, safe and effective ways to reduce weight, development of effective oral medications, the reasons for high rates of diabetes in certain ethnic populations, and ways to increase tissue sensitivity to insulin.

For all types of diabetes, topics of research include understanding the cause of complications and the best ways to treat these problems, developing new insulins and alternative methods of insulin delivery (e.g., oral, nasal, eye drops), new techniques for blood glucose monitoring, and the functions of somatostatin and glucagon. Some of these are discussed here.

BLOOD GLUCOSE MONITORING

For patients with diabetes, one of the most distressing aspects of managing the disorder on a daily basis is the need to prick a finger to obtain a sample of blood for assessing blood glucose levels. Periodically, the media report that a noninvasive glucose monitor has been developed that does not require pricking the finger. Although no such monitor is yet available for purchase, several companies are developing these devices, and some models are already in clinical trials.

The "Dream Beam®" is portable and can be held in one hand. It uses infrared light to measure the concentration of glucose. The user inserts a finger into the instrument, and the glucose reading is displayed in a window on the monitor. The device is battery powered and is durable and designed to last several years. The manufacturer states that test strips will not be required and that the overall cost will probably be less than that of currently used monitoring systems.

The "Glucowatch®" will allow patients to monitor blood glucose levels by pressing a button on the side of the watch. The watch uses electroosmosis to measure glucose levels every half hour.

Another company is developing a sensor that would be worn like an insulin pump and continuously monitor blood glucose levels. The device would warn the wearer through an audible alarm if glucose levels were too high or too low. One of the companies which makes an insulin pump has recently introduced a continuous glucose monitor. This device will be taken to the physicians office for download and will allow for more exacting adjustment of insulin. The long-term goal is to develop a sensor that would activate an insulin pump to deliver the appropriate amount of insulin in response to blood glucose levels.

GOOD DIABETES CONTROL

Does good control of blood glucose levels make a difference in the development of complications of diabetes? This question has been debated for several years. Many of the professionals who work in the field of diabetes and many patients who have diabetes would answer this question with an unequivocal yes. They have seen that patients who have good blood glucose levels feel better, look better, and have fewer acute

and long-term complications. Yet, studies done in the past (some with questionable validity) have never been able to concretely show that good diabetes control makes a difference.

The Diabetes Control and Complications Trial, a multicenter, 10-year, randomized clinical trial, was designed to determine the relationship between blood glucose control and early vascular complications of diabetes in patients with type 1 diabetes. The trial was concluded in 1993. The results were astoundingly conclusive: good blood glucose control significantly reduced the development of microvascular complications of diabetes (see chapter 8). The results were achieved by patients who had an average blood glucose level of 155 mg/dl and an HgbA1c concentration of 7.2%. An increase in the number of hypoglycemic episodes occurred, and these patients had undesired weight gain.

Only subjects with type 1 diabetes were included in the study. Thus, it is not known if these results also apply to patients with type 2 diabetes. The DCCT Research Group (1993) states that the microvascular, atherosclerotic, and neuropathic complications in type 1 and type 2 diabetes appear to be the same physiologically and that it is reasonable to think that control of blood glucose levels will also prevent or slow the progression of complications in type 2 diabetes.

The United Kingdom Prospective Study being carried out in England was a study done on over 5,000 individuals with newly diagnosed type 2 diabetes over a ten year period. It showed that even a modest reduction in blood glucose levels on a glycosylated hemoglobin test, was associated with a 35% reduction in retinopathy, nephropathy and neuropathy and with a 25% reduction in diabetes related death.

Another study on the effect of tight blood glucose control is being conducted by the Veterans Affairs hospitals. This study is known as the

Cooperative Study on Glycemic Control and Complications in type 2 diabetes (Whitehouse, 1992). Currently, a feasibility study is being done. If the results are suitable, it will be followed by a full-scale study to compare the effects of conventional diabetes control with those of intensive management of diabetes on cardiovascular complications of diabetes.

PREVENTING TYPE 1 DIABETES

Every year, type 1 diabetes develops in approximately 14,000 people. This type of diabetes is 20–50 times more likely to develop in first-degree relatives of people with diabetes than in those without diabetes. The process leading to type 1 diabetes begins months to years before the disease actually occurs. Two major methods of preventing type 1 diabetes are being investigated.

Autoimmunity

Autoimmunity is an important topic of interest in diabetes. The normal immune response helps the body fight against adverse effects caused by bacteria, viruses, or foreign substances. It provides the body with the ability to survive illnesses and infections. However, an overactive immune system may be responsible for the development of diabetes.

It is now possible to predict type 1 diabetes through detection of antibodies to islet cells, the GAD antibody, and antibodies to insulin (Bohannon, 1992). The assays are expensive, however, and it is not practical to test the entire population. The tests are currently being done at the University of Colorado in Denver, the University of Miami, and the University of California at Davis on first-degree relatives (mother, father, brother, sister, or child) of patients with type 1 diabetes. So far, the antibodies have been detected in less than 2% of the subjects tested. It may be many years before diabetes develops in these subjects.

Subjects who have tested positive for the antibodies have an intravenous glucose tolerance test done to ascertain the amount of insulin the pancreas is producing and the rate at which production occurs (the "K" factor). Subjects who have lost half or more of their beta cell secretory capacity and are destined to become diabetic are eligible for protocols to try to prevent the development of diabetes.

Scientists have recently discovered proteins, called superantigens (SAG), that they believe are responsible for triggering an attack by the immune system. They feel that physiological stresses such as an infection or the increase in steroid hormones at puberty cause a retrovirus to produce these SAGs.

A variety of prevention protocols have been tried. Immunosuppressive drugs (cyclosporine, azathioprine, prednisone) have been used and have slowed down the immune system and reversed the development of diabetes. These drugs have many side effects and may also suppress the immune system's ability to combat infections and other diseases such as cancer. Insulin is also used prophylactically to "rest" the pancreas and prevent destruction of the beta cells. Two diabetes prevention trials, the European nicotinamide trial and the insulin therapy trial, were begun in 1995 to investigate the prophylactic use of insulin in preventing the development of diabetes.

Viruses

Another area of research focuses on viruses as a possible cause of diabetes. The most commonly suspected viral agent is mumps virus. Other possibilities are coxsackievirus B4 and the viruses that cause hepatitis, mononucleosis, German measles, influenza, and the common cold. If a link between type 1 diabetes and a virus or viruses can be found, it might be possible to develop a vaccine that can prevent this type of diabetes.

Studies are also being conducted to see if the cells of the pancreas can be regenerated. PharmaTerra Inc. has recently demonstrated that male albino rats had pancreas regeneration when administered an herbal remedy called ProBeta®.

TRANSPLANTS

Transplantation related to the pancreas began in 1996 and to date over 9,000 transplants have been performed. Over 1,000 people in the US undergo a pancreas or simultaneous pancreas/kidney transplant every year. Immunosuppressants are critical to survival after transplants, but harmful to the body since they suppress the immune system so that the donor organ won't be attacked or rejected by the body. Success rates are impressive. Eighty eight percent of those who received a pancreas/kidney transplant did not have to take insulin after one year. After five years, there is a 70% success rate (still produces insulin) for a pancreas and a 81.4% patient survival rate. The cost of a kidney/pancreas transplant is $120–150,000. The average cost of a pancreas transplant is $60–90,000. In addition the cost of immunosuppressive drugs is very high.

ARTIFICIAL PANCREAS

Research has shown that beta cells can be implanted in host tissue, such as muscle tissue (outside the pancreas), and still function effectively. The cells manufacture insulin and in response to changes in the concentration of glucose in the blood release the correct amount of insulin to control blood glucose levels. Two problems are associated with this research, tissue rejection and a moral issue, because the beta cells are taken from aborted fetuses. In order to overcome these problems, two areas are being examined.

One area is use of pork-derived islet cells and a "selective membrane" that prevents antibodies from entering and attacking the encapsulated beta cell tissue. Pork insulin is similar to human insulin and has been successfully used for many years. With this method, use of fetal tissue and immunosuppressive drugs is avoided.

Another group of researchers is working on islet cell encapsulation that would eliminate the need for immunosuppressive drugs. This method involves enclosing insulin-producing islet cells in a semipermeable membrane that allows small molecules such as glucose, insulin, and nutrients to pass through but prevents larger immune system molecules from entering.

THE IMPLANTABLE INSULIN PUMP

An insulin pump is not an artificial pancreas. It cannot sense the level of glucose in the blood and automatically adjust insulin levels (see chapter 4). However, use of an insulin pump does allow a more physiologic response to changes in the concentration of blood glucose.

Insulin delivered subcutaneously by an indwelling needle attached to a catheter (the currently used external insulin pump system) is absorbed more slowly than insulin given intravenously or intraperitoneally. The implantable insulin pump is inserted into the abdominal cavity in a relatively simple surgical procedure. With the pump, the insulin goes into the peritoneal cavity and has an effect on the blood glucose level within 5–10 minutes. The amount of insulin delivered is controlled by using a hand-held "communicator" or control device.

One of the biggest advantages of this method of delivering insulin is that insulin requirements are much lower. Researchers think that using less insulin is a big advantage, because evidence suggests that high levels of insulin in the bloodstream may be related to macrovascular damage and atherosclerosis.

The ultimate goal is to develop an implantable closed-loop pump system that measures blood glucose levels automatically and then releases insulin on the basis of these measurements. Such a system would imitate the healthy body's response to glucose.

INSULIN DELIVERY

Recently, several reports have been published on an insulin nasal spray, an oral dosage of insulin, and insulin patches. Studies are being done on all these delivery methods. Each method has some inherent problems. Researchers are attempting to find a way to encapsulate insulin so that it will not be destroyed by digestive enzymes. Absorption of insulin in the form of a nasal spray is variable, and this method of delivery will probably only be effective in supplementing, not replacing, insulin injections. The insulin patch is in the early stages of development.

The FDA has begun human clinical trials of the oral insulin formula made by Generex Biotechnology. Called Oralgen® in the US, the liquid insulin is taken with an aerosol applicator.

Two companies are conducting trials on a very long acting or basal insulin which would mean fewer injections with insulin lasting as long as 48 hours.

SUMMARY

Diabetes and its multiple manifestations sometimes have a way of making everyone feel as if he or she has lost control. Using the tools of knowledge, the nursing care process, the multiplicity of resources available, a sense of humor, and a large dose of empathy can provide the health care team the power to help patients and patients' families fit diabetes into their lives instead of forcing them to fit their lives into diabetes.

Make sure that the person with diabetes is the Number One Person on the diabetes management team. No one knows more about that particular case of diabetes than the person who lives with it daily. The degree to which a patient and his or her family is involved in making decisions about diabetes management will depend on how comfortable they are in that role and the degree to which the plan of care is followed. We all need the knowledge and skills to function independently. Nurses must be instrumental in fostering and encouraging independence as soon as the patient is ready. Some people may need a gentle nudge toward independence. Nurses should be ready to give that nudge and still hold out a hand in case a helping hand is needed.

EXAM QUESTIONS

CHAPTER 11
Questions 99–100

99. An advantage to using the implantable insulin pump is that it

   a. senses the level of glucose in the blood.

   b. acts as an artificial pancreas.

   c. decreases the requirements for insulin.

   d. affects the blood glucose levels immediately.

100. An example of a non-invasive method of blood glucose monitoring is the

   a. DCCT.

   b. GAD.

   c. Generex.

   d. Dream Beam.

This concludes the final examination. An answer key will be sent with your certificate so that you can determine which of your answers were correct and incorrect.

APPENDIX

RESOURCES FOR DIABETES CARE

Each of these organizations may have a local office or chapter. Consult the telephone book for location and local listing.

American Association of Diabetes Educators
444 N. Michigan Avenue, Suite 1240
Chicago, IL 60611-3901
Tel: (800) 338-DMED
www.aadenet.org

American Diabetes Association
1660 Duke Street, Alexandria, VA 22313
Tel: (800) 232-3472
www.diabetes.org

American Heart Association
7272 Greenville Avenue, Box 45
Dallas, TX 75231-4596
Tel: (800) 242-8721
www.americanheart.org

International Diabetes Center
3800 Park Nicollet Boulevard
Minneapolis, MN 55416-9963
Tel: (612) 993-3393
http://onhealthnetworkcompany.com.

International Diabetic Athletes Association
1647 West Bethany Home Road #B
Phoenix, AZ 85015
Tel: (602) 433-2113
www.diabetes-exercise.org

Joslin Diabetes Center
One Joslin Place, Boston, MA 02215
Tel: (800) 344-4501
www.joslinharvard.edu

Juvenile Diabetes Foundation International
120 Wall Street, New York, NY 10005
Tel: (800) 223-1138
www.jdf.org

Medic Alert Foundation
P.O Box 1009, Turlock, CA 95381-1009
Tel: (800) 432-5378
www.medicalert.org

National Association for the Visually Handicapped
3201 Balboa Street, San Francisco, CA 94121
Tel: (415) 221-3201
www.navh.org

National Diabetes Information Clearinghouse
Box NDIC, 9000 Rockville Pike
Bethesda, MD 20892
Tel: (302) 654-3327
www.healthteach.com

National Federation of the Blind
811 Cherry Street, Suite 309
Columbia, MO 65201
www.nfb.org

NEWSLETTERS AND MAGAZINES

The following feature articles of interest on diabetes-related topics and products.

Diabetes Forecast Magazine
American Diabetes Association, Inc.
1660 Duke Street, Alexandria, VA 22314
www.diabetes.org

Diabetes Self Management
P.O. Box 52890, Boulder, CO 80322-2890
Tel: (800) 234-0923
www.diabetes-self-mgmt.com

Diabetes Interview
Kings Publications
3715 Balboa Street, San Francisco, CA 94121
Tel: (800) 234-1218
www.diabetesworld.com

The Diabetic Traveler
PO Box 8223 RW
Stamford, CT 06905

Voice of the Diabetic
National Federation of the Blind
Diabetics Division
Ed Bryant, Editor
811 Cherry Street, Suite 309
Columbia, MO 85201
www.nfb.org/voice.html

GLOSSARY

Acetone: A chemical formed in the blood when the body uses fat instead of glucose (sugar) for energy.

Acidosis: Too much acid in the body. For a person with diabetes, too much acid can lead to diabetic ketoacidosis.

Adult-onset diabetes: Former term for non-insulin-dependent or type 2 diabetes.

Albuminuria: The presence of more than normal amounts of a protein called albumin in the urine. *See also* microalbuminuria.

Aldose reductase inhibitors: A class of drugs being studied as a way to prevent eye and nerve damage in people with diabetes. They are thought to help prevent the conversion of glucose to sorbitol. Too much sorbitol trapped in eye and nerve cells can damage these cells.

Alpha cell: A type of cell in the pancreas that makes and releases glucagon, which raises blood glucose levels.

Amino acid: The building blocks of proteins; the main material of the body's cells.

Antagonist: An agent that opposes or fights the action of another agent.

Antibodies: Proteins that the body makes to protect itself from foreign substances.

Antidiabetes Agents: Medications that exert an effect on the body to improve blood sugar control through various mechanisms.

Aspartame: A man-made sweetener used in place of sugar.

Autonomic neuropathy: A disease of the nerves affecting the internal organs such as the bladder muscles, digestive tract, and genital organs.

Beta cell: A type of cell in the pancreas in areas called the islets of Langerhans that makes and releases insulin.

Blood glucose level: The amount of glucose in the bloodstream.

Blood glucose meter (or monitor): A small portable machine that determines how much sugar or glucose is in the blood by testing a sample of capillary blood.

Borderline diabetes: A term no longer used. See Impaired glucose tolerance.

Certified Diabetes Educator (CDE): A health care professional who is qualified by the American Association of Diabetes Educators to teach people with diabetes how to manage the disorder.

C peptide: The connecting link in the insulin molecule. Measurement of C peptide levels shows how much insulin the body is making.

Calorie: Energy that comes from food.

Capillary: The smallest of the body's blood vessels. Capillaries have walls so thin that oxygen and glucose can pass through and enter the cells.

Carbohydrates: Mainly sugars and starches that the body breaks down into glucose. The body also uses carbohydrates to make a substance called glycogen that is stored in the liver and muscles for future use.

Creatinine: A breakdown product of protein. Assays of the amount of creatinine are used to determine kidney functioning.

Cyclamate: A man-made chemical used in place of sugar. It was banned by the Food and Drug Administration in 1973 because research showed a link between use of cyclamate and an increase in the rates of bladder cancer.

Dawn phenomenon: A sudden increase in blood glucose levels in the early morning hours due to hormonal stimulation.

Dehydration: Great loss of body water. In a person with diabetes, an extremely high level of glucose causes osmotic diuresis and results in dehydration.

Delta cell: A type of cell in the pancreas, in the islets of Langerhans, that makes somatostatin.

Diabetes insipidus: A disease of the pituitary gland characterized by large urinary output.

Diabetic coma: A severe emergency in which a person is unconscious because of high blood glucose levels.

Diabetic ketoacidosis (DKA): Severe, out-of-control diabetes that requires emergency treatment. DKA occurs when not enough insulin is present. The body starts using stored fats for energy, and ketone bodies (acids) build up in the blood.

Diabetic retinopathy: A disease of the small blood vessels of the retina of the eye.

Diabetogenic: Causing diabetes. Certain drugs and some viruses may be diabetogenic.

Dialysis: A method of removing wastes from the blood when the kidneys no longer function properly. There are two types: hemodialysis and peritoneal dialysis.

Dietitian: An expert in nutrition who helps people learn about diet and meal planning.

Edema: A swelling or puffiness of some part of the body due to fluid retention.

Endocrine glands: Glands that release hormones into the bloodstream. The pancreas is an endocrine gland.

Endogenous: Grown or made inside the body. Insulin made by a person's own pancreas is endogenous. Injected insulin is exogenous.

Enzyme: A special type of protein that facilitates a chemical process.

Epinephrine: One of the secretions of the adrenal glands. It promotes release of glucose by the liver and limits the release of insulin. It also increases heart rate and blood pressure. Also called adrenalin.

Euglycemia: A normal level of glucose in the blood.

Exchange lists: A food grouping system used to help plan meals. There are six food groups: starch/bread, meat, vegetables, fruit, milk, and fats. Within a food group, each serving has about the same amount of carbohydrate, protein, fat, and calories.

Fructose: A type of sugar found in many fruits and vegetables and in honey.

Funduscopy: A method of looking at the back area of the eye to see if there is damage to the vessels that supply the retina.

Gastroparesis: A form of autonomic neuropathy that affects the stomach. Food is not digested properly and does not move through the stomach in a normal way, resulting in delayed gastric emptying and delayed glucose absorption.

Gestational diabetes mellitus (GDM): A type of diabetes mellitus that has its first occurrence in pregnancy. The blood glucose levels return to normal in about 95% of cases.

Glaucoma: An eye disease associated with increased intraocular pressure.

Glucagon: A hormone that increases the level of glucose in the bloodstream. In emergencies due to low levels of blood glucose, glucagon can be injected if the person affected cannot take sugar by mouth.

Glucose: The main sugar that the body makes from the three elements of food-proteins, fats, and carbohydrates-but mainly from carbohydrates. Glucose is the major source of energy for living cells and is carried to each cell through the bloodstream. The cells cannot use glucose without the help of insulin.

Glycemic response: The effect of different foods on blood glucose levels over time. Some kinds of foods may increase blood glucose levels more than other foods containing the same amount of carbohydrates.

Glycogen: The chief source of stored fuel in the body.

Glycosuria: The presence of glucose (sugar) in the urine.

Glycosylated hemoglobin/hemoglobin A1c (HgbA1c) test: A blood test that indicates what a person's average blood glucose (sugar) level was in the 2–3 months preceding the test.

HLA: Human lymphocyte antigen; proteins on the outer part of the cell that help the body fight illness. Scientists think that people with a certain type of HLA are more likely to have insulin-dependent diabetes.

Home blood glucose monitoring/self blood glucose monitoring: The method of testing capillary blood samples to determine the level of glucose in the bloodstream. It is very useful in helping patients carry out self-management of diabetes.

Hyperglycemia: Too high a level of glucose (sugar) in the blood.

Hyperinsulinemia: Too high a level of insulin in the blood. This can make a person have low concentrations of blood glucose.

Hyperlipidemia: Too high a level of fats (lipids) in the blood.

Hyperosmolar coma: A coma related to high levels of glucose in the blood that requires emergency treatment. The person affected is usually older and weak from loss of body fluids and weight. Ketones are not present or are present in very small amounts. Also called HHNK or HONK.

Hypoglycemia: Too low a level of glucose (sugar) in the blood.

Immunosuppressive drugs: Drugs that block or suppress the body's immune response.

Impaired glucose tolerance (IGT): Blood glucose levels higher than normal but below the level of those diagnostic for diabetes. Formerly called borderline or subclinical diabetes.

Insulin: A hormone that helps the body use glucose (sugar) for energy. Secreted by the beta cells of the pancreas located in the islets of Langerhans.

Insulin-dependent diabetes mellitus (IDDM): A chronic condition in which the pancreas makes little or no insulin. IDDM usually occurs in children and adults who are less than 30 years old. Insulin injections are necessary for life. Formerly called juvenile diabetes or ketosis-prone diabetes. It is now also called type 1 diabetes.

Insulin reaction: Too low a level of glucose (sugar) in the blood (hypoglycemia). Also called insulin shock.

Ketoacidosis: *See* Diabetic ketoacidosis

Ketones: One of the by-products of the breakdown of fat for energy when the body cannot use glucose for fuel because of a lack of insulin.

Kussmaul's breathing or respiration: The rapid, deep, and labored breathing of people who have ketoacidosis.

Labile diabetes: A term used to indicate when a person's blood glucose level often swings quickly from high to low and from low to high. Often caused by poor diabetes management. Also called brittle diabetes.

Lactic acidosis: The buildup of lactic acid in the body. A potentially fatal situation requiring immediate emergency attention.

Lipoatrophy: Small dents in the skin that can form when injection technique is poor or injections are made repeatedly in the same site. Much less prevalent with human insulins than with animal insulins.

Lipodystrophy: Lumps in the skin that can form when injection technique is poor or injections are made repeatedly in the same site. Much less prevalent with human insulins than with animal insulins.

Macrovascular disease: Disease of the large blood vessels. One of the causes is long-term diabetes with poor blood glucose control.

Maturity-onset diabetes: Term formerly used for non-insulin-dependent or type 2 diabetes.

Mauriac syndrome: A manifestation of long-term poor glucose control due to underinsulinization. It is characterized by growth retardation, sexual infantilism with delayed puberty, hyperlipidemia, a round face, a protuberant abdomen, and hepatomegaly.

Metabolism: The term for the way cells chemically change food so it can be used by the body.

mg/dl: The abbreviation for milligrams per deciliter or tenth of a liter. Used as the unit of measure for blood glucose levels.

Microalbuminuria: The presence of small amounts of albumin in the urine. Often the first laboratory evidence of kidney damage. *See also* albuminuria.

Microvascular disease: A disease of the small blood vessels of the body. In diabetes the triopathy of diabetes microvascular diseases is retinopathy (eye disease), neuropathy (nerve disease), and nephropathy (kidney disease).

Non-insulin-dependent diabetes mellitus (NIDDM): The most common form of diabetes mellitus. Usually occurs in people more than 40 years old who are overweight and have a strong family history of this type of diabetes. Formerly called adult-onset, maturity-onset, or ketosis-resistant diabetes. It is now also called type 2 diabetes.

Obesity: An increase in body weight beyond the amount required for a person's size and age that is due to excessive fat; the state of having body fat that is 20% or more than that considered normal for age.

Oral hypoglycemic agents (OHAs): Pills taken to lower the amount of glucose in the blood. They are not insulin but may cause low blood sugar reactions due to their mechanism of action.

Pancreas: An organ behind the lower part of the stomach that is about the size of a hand. The cells in the pancreas produce insulin, glucagon, and somatostatin.

Periodontal disease: Damage to the gums that can result in tooth loss. Poor diabetes control can contribute to this disease.

Peripheral vascular disease: Disease of the blood vessels of the arms, legs, and feet.

Pharmaceutic action: The pharmokinetic duration of action. The action of insulin on entrance into and exit from the body.

Polydipsia: Excessive thirst. A classic symptom of diabetes.

Polyphagia: Excessive hunger. A classic symptom of diabetes.

Polyuria: Excessive urination. A classic sign of diabetes.

Proinsulin: The precursor of insulin. Proinsulin is made in the pancreas and then converted to insulin. When insulin is purified from pork or beef pancreata, the proinsulin is not fully removed. The remaining amount can cause rashes, insulin resistance, lipoatrophy, and lipodystrophy.

Receptors: Areas on the outer part of a cell that allow the cell to join or bind with insulin.

Renal threshold: The level at which the blood-stream is holding the maximum amount of glucose. At levels greater than the threshold, glucose spills over into the urine.

Risk factor: Anything that increases the chance that a person will get a disease.

Secondary diabetes: Diabetes caused by or associated with another disease or due to taking certain drugs or chemicals.

SMBG: Self monitoring of blood glucose by the individual or caregiver for the person with diabetes using a glucose meter designed for home use.

Somatostatin: A hormone made by the delta cells of the pancreas in the islets of Langerhans. It may control how the body secretes two other hormones, insulin and glucagon.

Somogyi effect: A swing to high levels of glucose (sugar) in the blood from an extremely low level. It usually occurs after an untreated insulin reaction during the night.

Sorbitol: A sugar alcohol the body uses slowly. It is a nutritive sweetener, because it has four calories in every gram. Sorbitol is also produced by the body. Too much sorbitol in the cells can cause damage. Diabetic retinopathy and neuropathy may be related to too much sorbitol in the cells of the eyes and nerves.

Split dose: Division of a prescribed daily dose of insulin into two or more injections given over the course of a day.

Therapeutic Action: Effective duration of action. The amount of active insulin needed to keep blood glucose levels in normal limits.

Triglyceride: A type of body fat. The body needs insulin to remove this type of fat from the blood.

Type 1 diabetes mellitus: Diabetes that requires the replacement of insulin or insulin dependent diabetes.

Type 2 diabetes mellitus: Diabetes that occurs usually later in life and is directly related to family history, obesity and sedentary lifestyle. Treatment may include oral medications and insulin if diet and exercise do not control blood sugars.

Uremia: A symptom of end stage renal disease that develops as renal function declines and urea, creatinine and other metabolic wastes accumulate in the blood.

Vitrectomy: Surgical removal of the clear gel that fills the center of the eye. Used when blood and scar tissue are present. The surgeon replaces the gel with clear fluid.

BIBLIOGRAPHY

Aiello, L. & Cavallerano, J. (1991). Ocular complications. In H. Lebovitz (Ed.), *Therapy for Diabetes Mellitus and related disorders.* Alexandria, VA: American Diabetes Association.

Aiello, L. M., Rand, L. I., Briones, J. C., Wafai, M. Z. & Sebestyen, J. G. (1981). Diabetic retinopathy in Joslin Clinic patients with adult-onset diabetes. *Ophthalmology, 88*(7), 619–623.

Alberti, K. (1990). Diabetes and surgery. In M. Ellenberg & H. Rifkin (Eds.), *Diabetes Mellitus: Theory and practice* (4th ed.). New Hyde Park, NY: Medical Examination Publishing.

American Association of Diabetes Educators (Oct. 1998). *Core curriculum for diabetes educators.* Wichita: University of Kansas, School of Medicine.

American Diabetes Association (1985). Proceedings of the second international work-shop-conference on gestational Diabetes Mellitus. *Diabetes, 34*(Suppl. 2), 1–130.

American Diabetes Association, Inc. (1998). *Exchange lists for meal planning* (p. 22).

American Diabetes Association (1999). Clinical practice recommendations, 1999. *Diabetes Care, 22*(Suppl. 1), 1–114.

Amylin Pharmaceuticals Incorporated (1998). *Physiology of Glycemic Control.*

Anderson, J. & Campbell, K. (1990). Mixing insulins in 1990. *The Diabetes Educator, 16,* 5.

Arauz-Pacheco, C. & Raskin, P. (1991). Surgery and anesthesia. In H. Lebovitz (Ed.), *Therapy for Diabetes Mellitus and related disorders.* Alexandria, VA: American Diabetes Association.

Bailey, C. J. (1992). Biguanides and NIDDM. *Diabetes Care, 15*(6), 755–772.

Benson, J. (1985). Disorders of carbohydrate metabolism. In R. Metz, & E. Larson (Eds.), *Blue book of endocrinology.* Philadelphia: Saunders.

Benz, M. M. & Kohler, E. (1980). Baby food exchanges and feeding the diabetic infant. *Diabetes Care, 3*(4), 554–556.

Bernstein, R. (1981). Diabetes: The Glucograf method for normalizing blood sugar. In *The Joslin diabetes manual.* Philadelphia: Lea & Febiger.

Betschart, J. (1992). Americans with Disabilities Act: New job rights for the disabled. *The Diabetes Educator, 18*(4).

Betz, J. (1995). Fast acting insulin analogs: A promising innovation in diabetes control. *The Diabetes Educator, 21*(3).

Bingham, P. & Riddle, M. (1989). Combined insulin-sulfonylurea treatment of type II diabetes. *The Diabetes Educator, 15*(5).

Bohannon, N. (1992). Keep your children from getting diabetes: Dr. Nancy Bohannon talks about preventing type I diabetes. *Diabetes Interview, 2, 3.*

Bolognia, J. & Braverman, I. (1991). In H. Lebovitz (Ed.), *Therapy for Diabetes Mellitus and related disorders*. Alexandria, VA: American Diabetes Association.

Brodows, R. (1998). Repaglinide (Prandin): A new therapy for type 2 diabetes. *Practical Diabetology, 6,* 32–36.

Bryant, E. (1992). "Dream Beam": Not just a dream anymore. *Diabetes Interview, 2, 2.*

Buchanan, T., Unterman, T. & Metzger, B. (1985). The medical management of diabetes in pregnancy. *Clinics in Perinatology, 12*(3), 625–650.

California Diabetes and Pregnancy Program. *Guidelines for care* (p. 207).

Campbell, K. (1988, July/August). Practical pharmacology: Human insulin. *Practical Diabetology.*

Campbell, K. (1989). *Diabetes and the pharmacist* (3rd ed.). West Haven, CT: Diagnostics Division, Miles Inc.

Chase, H. P., Jackson, W. E., Hooks, S. L., Cockerham, R. S., Archer, P. G. & O'Brien, D. (1989). Glucose control and the renal and retinal complications of insulin-dependent diabetes. *Journal of the American Medical Association, 261*(8), 1155–1160.

Christensen, M. H., Funnell, M. M., Ehrlich, M. R., Fellows, E. P. & Floyd, J. C. (1991). How to care for the diabetic foot. *American Journal of Nursing, 91*(3), 50–56.

Connell, F. A., Vadheim, C. & Emanuel, I. (1985). Diabetes in pregnancy: A population-based study of incidence, referral for care, and perinatal mortality. *American Journal of Obstetrics and Gynecology, 151*(5), 598–603.

Controlling type II diabetes through meal planning and exercise (1985). Daly City, CA: Krames Communications.

Coustan, D. (1991). Gestational diabetes. In H. Lebovitz (Ed.), *Therapy for Diabetes Mellitus and related disorders*. Alexandria, VA: American Diabetes Association.

Cox, D. J., Taylor, A. G., Nowacek, G., Holley-Wilcox, P. & Pohl, S. L. (1984). The relationship between psychological stress and insulin-dependent diabetic blood glucose control: Preliminary investigations. *Health Psychology, 3.*

Cryer, P. E., White, N. H. & Santiago, J. V. (1986). The relevance of glucose counterregulatory systems to patients with insulin-dependent Diabetes Mellitus. *Endocrine Reviews, 7*(2), 131–139.

Davidson, J. (1986). *Clinical Diabetes Mellitus: A problem-oriented approach.* New York: Thieme.

Davidson, M. (1998). *Diagnosis and treatment* (4th Ed.). Philadelphia: WB Saunders.

DeFronzo, R. (1991). In H. Lebovitz (Ed.), *Therapy for Diabetes Mellitus and related disorders.* Alexandria, VA: American Diabetes Association.

Diabetes Control and Complications Trial (DCCT) Research Group (1993). The effect of intensive treatment of diabetes on the development and progression of long-term complications in insulin-dependent Diabetes Mellitus. *New England Journal of Medicine, 392*(14), 977–986.

Diabetic Retinopathy Study Research Group (1979). Report no. 3: Four risk factors for visual loss in diabetic retinopathy. *Archives of Ophthalmology, 97*(4), 654–655.

Early Treatment Diabetic Retinopathy Study Research Group (1985). Photocoagulation for diabetic macular edema: Early treatment diabetes retinopathy study report no. 1. *Archives of Ophthalmology, 103*(12), 1796–1806.

Eckerling, L. & Kohrs, M. B. (1984). Research on compliance with diabetic regimens: Applications to practice. *Journal of the American Dietetic Association, 84*(7), 805–809.

Edeleman, S. & Kruger, D. (1997). A new look at glucose control. *Practical Diabetology, 12,* 9–13.

Eisenbarth, G. S. (1986). Type I diabetes mellitus: A chronic autoimmune disease. *New England Journal of Medicine, 314*(21), 1360–1368.

Ellenberg, M. & Rifkin, H. (1983). *Diabetes Mellitus: Theory and practice* (3rd ed.). New Hyde Park, NY: Medical Examination Publishing.

Franz, M. J. (1985). *Diabetes and exercise: Guidelines for safe and enjoyable activity.* International Diabetes Center.

Freinkel, N. (1980). Gestational diabetes 1979: Philosophical and practical aspects to a major health problem. *Diabetes Care, 3*(3), 399–401.

Fritz, M. & Offenbacher, S. (1986). Oral disorders in Diabetes Mellitus. In J. Davidson, *Clinical Diabetes Mellitus: A problem-oriented approach.* New York: Thieme.

Funnell, M. et al. (1998). *A core curriculum for diabetes education* (3rd ed.). Chicago: American Association of Diabetes Educators.

Gale, E. A. M., Dornan, T. L. & Tatersall, R. B. (1981). Severely uncontrolled diabetes in the over-fifties. *Diabetologia, 21*(1), 25–28.

Genuth, S. (1991). Diabetic ketoacidosis and hyperglycemic hyperosmolar coma in adults. In H. Lebovitz (Ed.), *Therapy for Diabetes Mellitus and related disorders.* Alexandria, VA: American Diabetes Association.

Gibbons, G. & Logerfo, F. (1991). Foot ulcers and infections. In H. Lebovitz (Ed.), *Therapy for Diabetes Mellitus and related disorders.* Alexandria, VA: American Diabetes Association.

Gilgor, R. & Lazarus, G. (1981). Skin manifestations of Diabetes Mellitus. In H. Rifkin & P. Raskin (Eds.), *Diabetes Mellitus.* Bowie, MD: F. J. Brady.

Glycosylated hemoglobin (1983). Calabasas Hills, CA: Endocrine Sciences.

Guthrie, H. (1986). *Introductory nutrition.* St. Louis: Mosby.

Harris, M. & Entmacher, P. (1985). Mortality from diabetes. In M. Harris & R. Hamman (Eds.), *Diabetes in America* (NIH Publication No. 85-1468). Washington, DC: U.S. Government Printing Office.

Harris, M. I., Hadden, W. C., Knowler, W. C., Bennett, P. A. (1987). Prevalence of diabetes and impaired glucose tolerance and plasma glucose levels in U.S. population aged 20–74 years. *Diabetes, 36*(4), 523–534.

Hazlett, J. (1993). *The diabetes control and complications trial: Diabetes self-management.*

Holcomb, J. (1995). *Storage of insulin.* Indianapolis: Eli Lilly Research Laboratories.

Holmes, D. M. (1986). The person and diabetes in psychosocial context. *Diabetes Care, 9*(2), 194–206.

Holmes, T. M. & Rahe, R. H. (1967). The social readjustment rating scale. *Psychosomatic Research, 11,* 213–218.

Jaffe, D., Orioli, E. & Scott, C. (1984). *Stress map.* San Francisco: Essi Systems.

James, R. C. & Chase, G. R. (1974). Evaluation of some commonly used semiquantitative methods for urinary glucose and ketone determinations. *Diabetes, 23*(5), 474–479.

Jacober, S. (1998). Insulin therapy and combination regimens for type 2 diabetes. *Practical Dermatology, 6,* 17–24.

Joslin, E. P. (1959). The treatment of diabetes mellitus. In E. Joslin, H. Root, P. White & A. Marble (Eds.), *Treatment of Diabetes Mellitus* (10th ed.). Philadelphia: Lea and Febiger.

Jovanovic, L. et al. (1982). The management of diabetes and pregnancy. In C. Peterson (Ed.), *Diabetes management in the '80s.* New York: PW Communications.

Jovanovic-Peterson, L. (1994, May). When to start insulin in the gestational diabetic. *Diabetes Professional.*

Kannel, W. & McGee, D. L. (1979). Diabetes and cardiovascular risk factors: The Framingham Study. *Circulation, 59*(1), 8–13.

Keen, H. & Jarrett, R. J. (1979). The WHO multinational study of vascular disease in diabetes: Macrovascular disease prevalence. *Diabetes Care, 2*(2), 187–195.

King, S. (1995). Watch development progressing smoothly. *Diabetes Interview, 40*(11).

King, S. (1997). Islet cell transplant update. In *Diabetes Interview, 65*(12), 1–21.

King, S. (1996b). Minimed's indwelling glucose sensor. *Diabetes Interview, 43*(2).

Krall, L. & Beaser, R. (1989). *Joslin diabetes manual.* Philadelphia: Lea & Febiger.

Kubler-Ross, E. (1970). *On death and dying.* New York: Macmillan.

Kulkarni, K. D. (1987). Altering the basic meal plan. In M. Power (Ed.), *Handbook of diabetes nutritional management* (pp. 187–188). Rockville, MD: Aspen.

Lammers, C. A., Naliboff, B. D. & Straatmeyer, A. J. (1984). The effects of progressive relaxation on stress and diabetic control. *Behavior Research and Therapy, 22*(6), 641–650.

Leahy, M. (1985). *Depression in adult insulin-dependent diabetes.* Dissertation, University of Kansas School of Medicine, Wichita.

Learning to live well with diabetes (1987). DCI Publishing.

Lebovitz, H. (Ed.) (1991). *Therapy for Diabetes Mellitus and related disorders.* Alexandria, VA: American Diabetes Association.

Levin, M. (1991). Peripheral arterial disease and intermittent claudication. In H. Lebovitz (Ed.), *Therapy for Diabetes Mellitus and related disorders.* Alexandria, VA: American Diabetes Association.

Lipson, L. G. (1985). Diabetes in the elderly: Diagnosis, pathogenesis, and therapy. *American Journal of Medicine, 80*(5A), 10–21.

Little, D. & Carnevali, D. (1976). *Nursing care planning* (2nd ed.). Philadelphia: Lippincott.

Lodewick, P. (1988). *A diabetic doctor looks at diabetes: His and yours.* Waltham, MA: RMI Corporation.

National Diabetes Education Initiative (1998). *Issues in Type 2 Diabetes, 2*(3)1–4.

National Society to Prevent Blindness (1980). *Vision problems in the United States: Data analysis.* New York: Author.

Nelson, R. (1990). The oral glucose tolerance test in clinical practice. *Practical Diabetology, 9,* 1.

Olson, O. (1988). *Diagnosis and management of Diabetes Mellitus.* New York: Raven.

Palmberg, P., Smith, M., Waltman, S., Krupin T., Singer P., Burgess D., Wendtlant T., Achtenberg J., Cryer P., Santiago J., White N., Kilo C. & Daughaday W. (1980). The natural history of retinopathy in insulin-dependent juvenile-onset diabetes. *Ophthalmology, 88*(7), 613–618.

Parke-Davis Professional Communication (1998). *Important drug warning related to use of Rezulin.*

Pederson, J. & Molsted-Pederson, L. (1965). Prognosis of the outcome of pregnancies in diabetics: A new classification. *Acta Endocrinologica, 50,* 70–78.

Pfeifer, M. (1991). Cardiac denervation syndrome. In H. Lebovitz (Ed.), *Therapy for Diabetes Mellitus and related disorders.* Alexandria, VA: American Diabetes Association.

Pickup, J. & Williams, G. (Eds.) (1991). *Textbook of diabetes.* Oxford, England: Blackwell Scientific.

Pirart, J. (1977). Diabetes Mellitus and its degenerative complications: A prospective study of 4,400 patients observed between 1947 and 1973. *Diabete et Metabolisme, 3*(4), 245–256.

Pollack, H. (1953). Stanley Rossiter Benedict: Creator of laboratory tests for glycosuria. *Diabetes, 2*(5), 420–421.

Powers, M. (Ed.) (1996). *Handbook of diabetes nutritional management.* Rockville, MD: Aspen.

Reece, E. & Quintero, R. (1991). In H. Lebovitz (Ed.), *Therapy for Diabetes Mellitus and related disorders.* Alexandria, VA: American Diabetes Association.

Reichel, W. (Ed.) (1995). *Care of the elderly: Clinical aspects of aging.* Baltimore: Williams & Wilkins.

Rifkin, H. (Ed.) (1985). *The physician's guide to type II diabetes (NIDDM): Diagnosis and treatment.* Alexandria VA: American Diabetes Association.

Rosenbaum, L. (1983). Biofeedback-assisted stress management for insulin-treated Diabetes Mellitus. *Biofeedback and Self Regulation, 8*(4), 519–532.

Rosling, B. G., Slots, J., Christersson, L. A. & Genco, R. J. (1982). Topical chemical antimicrobial therapy in the management of the subgingival microflora and periodontal disease. *Journal of Periodontal Research, 17*(5), 541–543.

Ross, H., Berstein, G. & Rifkin, H. (1983). Relationship of metabolic control of Diabetes Mellitus to long-term complications. In M. Ellenberg & H. Rifkin, *Diabetes Mellitus: Theory and practice,* (pp. 363–372). New Hyde Park, NY: Medical Examination Publishing.

Rudolf, M. C. J., Coustan, D. R., Sherwin, R.S., Bates S. E., Felig, P., Genel, M. & Tamborlane, W. V. (1981). Efficacy of the insulin pump in the home treatment of pregnant diabetics. *Diabetes, 30*(11), 891–895.

Santiago, J. et al. (1991). Hypoglycemia in patients with type I diabetes. In H. Lebovitz (Ed.), *Therapy for Diabetes Mellitus and related disorders,* (pp. 211–236). Alexandria, VA: American Diabetes Association.

Sattley, M. (1998). Has the pancreas transplant come of age? The facts and fiction. *Diabetes Interview,* 71.

Schwartz, S. (1991). *Management of Diabetes Mellitus.* Durant, OK: Essential Medical Systems.

Selye, H. (1957). *The stress of life.* London: Longmans, Green.

Sinnock, P. (1985). Hospital utilization for diabetes. In M. Harris, & R. Hamman (Eds.), *Diabetes in America* (NIH Publication No. 85-1468). Washington, DC: U.S. Government Printing Office.

Sowers, J. (1991). In H. Lebovitz (Ed.), *Therapy for Diabetes Mellitus and related disorders.* Alexandria, VA: American Diabetes Association.

Sperling, M. (Ed.) (1988). *The physician's guide to insulin-dependent (type I) diabetes: Diagnosis and treatment.* Alexandria VA: American Diabetes Association.

Stein, R., Goldberg, N., Kalman, F.l. & Chesler, R. (1984). Exercise and the patient with type I Diabetes Mellitus. *Pediatric Clinics of North America, 31*(3), 665–673.

Strand, C. & Ehrenkranz, R. (1991). Infants of diabetic mothers. In H. Lebovitz (Ed.), *Therapy for Diabetes Mellitus and related disorders.* Alexandria, VA: American Diabetes Association.

Sullivan, B. (1979). Adjustment in diabetic adolescent girls: II. Adjustment, self-esteem, and depression in diabetic adolescent girls. *Psychosomatic Medicine, 41*(2), 127–138.

Upjohn Company (1992). *Drug information bulletin.* Kalamazoo, MI: Author.

UK Prospective Diabetes Study (UKDPS) Group (1998). Intensive blood-glucose control with sulphonylureas or insulin compared with conventional treatment and risk of complications in patients with type 2 diabetes (UKDPS 33). *Lancet, 352,* 837–53.

Villeneuve, M., Treitel, L. & D'Eramo, G. (1985). Dental care for the person with Diabetes Mellitus. *The Diabetes Educator, 11*(3).

Yura, H. & Walsh, M. (1978). *The nursing process* (3rd ed.). New York: Appleton-Century-Crofts.

Waif, S. (Ed.) (1980). *Diabetes Mellitus.* Indianapolis: Eli Lilly.

Wason, C. & Metzger, B. (1986). *Diabetes management for mothers-to-be: You can do it.* Elkhart, IN: Ames Center for Diabetes Education.

White, N. H., Gingerich, R. L., Levandoski, L. A., Cryer, P. E. & Santiago, J. V. (1985). Plasma pancreatic polypeptide response to insulin-induced hypoglycemia as a marker for defective glucose counterregulation in insulin-dependent Diabetes Mellitus. *Diabetes, 34*(9), 870–875.

Whitehouse, F. (1992). Toward risk factor control for all patients with diabetes. *Diabetes Care, 15*(11), 1818–1820.

INDEX

PRETEST KEY

Diabetes Nursing Care:
Overview and Management

1.	c	Chapter 1
2.	d	Chapter 1
3.	b	Chapter 1
4.	a	Chapter 1
5.	a	Chapter 2
6.	d	Chapter 2
7.	c	Chapter 2
8.	d	Chapter 3
9.	a	Chapter 3
10.	d	Chapter 3
11.	d	Chapter 4
12.	a	Chapter 4
13.	c	Chapter 4
14.	b	Chapter 5
15.	d	Chapter 5
16.	b	Chapter 5
17.	c	Chapter 6
18.	b	Chapter 6
19.	b	Chapter 7
20.	a	Chapter 7
21.	b	Chapter 8
22.	c	Chapter 8
23.	c	Chapter 9
24.	b	Chapter 9
25.	c	Chapter 7

Notes

Notes

Notes

Notes

Notes

Notes

Western Schools® offers over 60 topics to suit all your interests – and requirements!

Clinical Conditions/Nursing Practice

A Nurse's Guide to Weight Control
    for Healthy Living...25 hrs
Airway Management with a Tracheal Tube ....1 hr
Auscultation Skills: Breath and Heart Sounds ......12 hrs
Basic Nursing of Head, Chest, Abdominal,
    Spine and Orthopedic Trauma ....16 hrs
Care at the End of Life..3 hrs
Chest Tube Management ....2 hrs
Death, Dying & Bereavement ....30 hrs
Diabetes Nursing Care ....30 hrs
Healing Nutrition ....24 hrs
Hepatitis C: The Silent Killer ....2 hrs
HIV/AIDS...................................1, 2, 4 or 30 hrs
Holistic & Complementary Therapies: Introduction..1 hr
Managing Obesity and Eating Disorders ....30 hrs
Nursing Care of the HIV-Infected Patient..............30 hrs
Orthopedic Nursing: Caring for Patients with
    Musculoskeletal Disorders ....30 hrs
Pain Management: Principles and Practice............30 hrs
The Neurological Exam..1 hr
Wound Management and Healing..........................30 hrs

Cosmetic Treatments/Surgery

Belt Lipectomy: Lower Body Contouring ....1 hr
Botox Treatments and Dermal Fillers.......................1 hr
Cosmetic Breast Surgery ....1 hr
Weight Loss Surgery ....1 hr

Critical Care/ER/OR

Ambulatory Surgical Care ....20 hrs
Case Studies in Critical Care Nursing: A Guide for
    Application and Review ....46 hrs
Principles of Basic Trauma Nursing ....30 hrs

Geriatrics

Alzheimer's Disease: A Complete Guide for Nurses ..25 hrs
Alzheimer's: Things a Nurse Needs to Know ......12 hrs
Elder Abuse ....4 hrs
Home Health Nursing ....30 hrs
Nursing Care of the Older Adult ....30 hrs
Psychosocial Issues Affecting Older Adults ....16 hrs

Infectious Diseases/Bioterrorism

Biological Weapons ....5 hrs
Bioterrorism & the Nurse's Response to WMD ......5 hrs
Bioterrorism Readiness: The Nurse's Critical Role .. 2 hrs
Infection Control Training for Healthcare Workers ..4 hrs
Influenza: A Vaccine-Preventable Disease ....1 hr
SARS: An Emerging Public Health Threat ....1 hr
Smallpox..2 hrs
The New Threat of Drug Resistant Microbes ....5 hrs
West Nile Virus ....1 hr

Oncology

Cancer in Women...30 hrs
Cancer Nursing: A Solid Foundation for Practice ..30 hrs
Chemotherapy Essentials: Principles & Practice ..15 hrs

Pediatrics/Maternal-Child/Women's Health

Attention Deficit Hyperactivity Disorders
    Throughout the Lifespan.................................30 hrs
Diabetes in Children ....30 hrs
End-of-Life Care for Children and
    Their Families ....2 hrs
Manual of School Health ....30 hrs
Maternal-Newborn Nursing..................................30 hrs
Menopause: Nursing Care for Women
    Throughout Mid-Life ....25 hrs
Pediatric Nursing: Routine to Emergent Care........30 hrs
Pediatric Pharmacology ....10 hrs
Pediatric Physical Assessment..............................10 hrs
Women's Health: Contemporary
    Advances and Trends ....30 hrs

Professional Issues/Management/Law

Medical Error Prevention: Patient Safety ....2 hrs
Nursing Practice and the Law ....30 hrs
Nursing and Malpractice Risks:
    Understanding the Law...................................30 hrs
Ohio Law: Standards of Safe Nursing Practice ....1 hr
Supervisory Skills for Nurses ....30 hrs
Surviving and Thriving in Nursing ....30 hrs
Understanding Managed Care ....30 hrs

Psychiatric/Mental Health

Basic Psychopharmacology...................................5 hrs
IPV (Intimate Partner Violence):
    A Domestic Violence Concern ....1 or 3 hrs
Psychiatric Principles & Applications for
    General Patient Care ....30 hrs
Psychiatric Nursing: Current Trends
    in Diagnosis and Treatment ....30 hrs
Substance Abuse ....30 hrs

Visit us online at www.westernschools.com for these great courses – plus all the latest CE topics!
Online testing also available.

REV. 1/20/05